Clinics in Developmental Medicine No. 89

OPTIC FUNDUS SIGNS OF DEVELOPMENTAL AND NEUROLOGICAL DISORDERS IN CHILDREN— A MANUAL FOR CLINICIANS

LOIS J. MARTYN
ANTHONY J. PILEGGI
HENRY W. BAIRD

1985
Spastics International Medical Publications
OXFORD: Blackwell Scientific Publications Ltd.
PHILADELPHIA: J. B. Lippincott Co.

© 1985 Spastics International Medical Publications
5a Netherhall Gardens, London NW3 5RN

First published 1985

British Library Cataloguing in Publication Data
Martyn, Lois J.
Optic fundus signs of developmental and neurological disorders in
children—(Clinics in developmental medicine; 89)
1. Pediatric neurology—Diagnosis
2. Physical diagnosis
I. Title II. Pileggi, Anthony J. III. Baird, Henry W. IV. Series.
618.92'804754   RJ488

ISBN 0-632-01292-7

Printed in Great Britain at
The Lavenham Press Ltd.,
Lavenham, Suffolk

CONTENTS

CONTRIBUTORS

LOIS J. MARTYN

Associate Professor of Ophthalmology and Associate Professor in Pediatrics, Temple University School of Medicine, Philadelphia; Pediatric Ophthalmologist, St. Christopher's Hospital for Children, Philadelphia.

ANTHONY J. PILEGGI

Professor of Pediatrics, Temple University School of Medicine, Philadelphia; Director, Handicapped Children's Unit, St. Christopher's Hospital for Children, Philadelphia.

HENRY W. BAIRD

Professor of Pediatrics, Emeritus, Temple University School of Medicine, Philadelphia.

FOREWORD

The ophthalmological study of the child's eye allows an unique opportunity for documenting puzzling fundus changes. This technique demonstrates an intimate relationship between fundus changes and abnormalities which help us interpret difficult and often frustrating problems in the developmental and neurological disorders of children. The explosive developments in genetics, metabolic diseases, immunology, pathology, neonatology and other fields, including bio-engineering and sophisticated diagnostic techniques, have served to increase our awareness of subtle fundus and other ocular changes, revealing the clues which help us with the diagnosis.

I recall a fundus examination carried out more than 30 years ago on a child admitted for the ninth time for seizures of unknown origin. A large, white, elevated lesion in the mid-periphery of the fundus was diagnosed as tuberous sclerosis, allowing an understanding of this child's neurological disorder for the first time.

In addition to pointing out the pathological processes which can be observed, the authors of this monograph have also helped to make us aware of the wide range of fundal variations in both the normal- and delayed-developing posterior pole and retinal-pigment layer. The gradual sorting-out of this valuable collection of teaching material has required devotion and a great deal of time and patience. I congratulate the authors for making this valuable contribution to developmental pediatrics and child neurology, since it represents a significant step in the documentation of the causal-related changes observable in the abnormally developing child. It is hoped that their careful observations will stimulate other astute observers to build on this information and to improve our interpretation and understanding of this important aspect of pediatric neurology.

R. D. Harley, M.D., Ph.D.
Attending Surgeon,
Wills Eye Hospital,
Philadelphia.
August 1984

PREFACE

The intent of the authors is to provide descriptions and brief discussions of optic fundus signs for use by students, residents in pediatrics and interested physicians. The book is written as a practical and useful guide for clinical evaluation. It is not an ophthalmological text, and detailed analyses are beyond its scope. We have included those conditons which we believe are of principal importance in caring for children with developmental and neurological disorders.

INTRODUCTION

Readily accessible for examination and subject to a wide range of developmental and pathological changes of both focal and systemic nature, the eyegrounds command special attention in the diagnosis of neurological disorders of childhood.

Of primary importance are the optic-nervehead signs of disease, such as papilledema, papillitis and optic atrophy, and a number of anomalies such as optic-nerve hypoplasia, aplasia and various colobomatous defects. Equally important are the retinal manifestations of neurological and systemic disease, including diffuse and focal chorioretinitis, the pigmentary retinal degenerations, a number of special maculopathies and the various retinal phakomata.

Essential to detection and proper interpretation of these signs are diligence and skill in the use of the ophthalmoscope, an appreciation of the range of variation in the appearance of the normal fundus, and an understanding of the ways in which pathological processes are manifested in the highly specialized tissues of the eye.

THE OPHTHALMOSCOPE

The standard, direct, hand-held ophthalmoscope consists basically of a source of light, devices to modify the projected beam of light, and a system of lenses to allow precise focusing of the image (Fig. 1).

Adequate light is important. Instruments that connect to house current *via* a transformer provide optimal light and are preferred by many clinicians. Most battery-operated ophthalmoscopes provide sufficient light for average clinical needs and are conveniently portable. However, the batteries must be kept well-charged, and the bulb should be replaced as often as necessary for optimal clarity. In both types, the intensity of the light can be controlled with a rheostat.

1

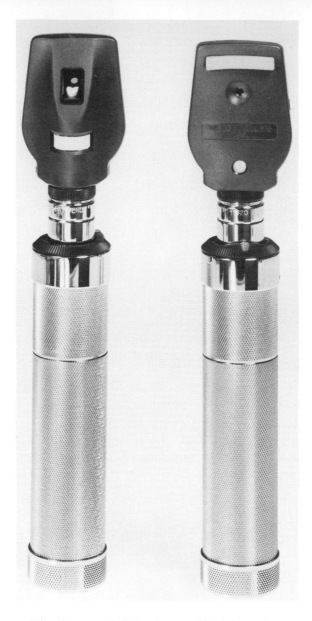

Figure 1.
The No. 11620 halogen co-axial ophthalmoscope from Welch Allyn. Photograph courtesy of Welch Allyn Inc., Skaneateles Falls, New York, USA.

The beam of light is modified by using the various apertures and accessories provided. In most instruments these include a small and a large round aperture, a vertical-slit aperture, a grid pattern and a red-free (green) filter. The small round aperture is used for viewing through a small pupil; the large round aperture for viewing through a large or dilated pupil. The vertical-slit aperture is intended for assessing the contour (convexity, concavity) of fundus lesions—elevated or depressed lesions produce bowing or step-like disruption of the slit-beam; flat lesions produce no distortion. The grid pattern can be used for gauging and recording the size of lesions or the caliber of vessels. The green lens or red-free light is used to help differentiate blood from pigment—blood (or old hemoglobin) appears dark black in red-free light, whereas melanin appears less black. The striations of the normal nerve-fiber pattern also are seen better in red-free light.

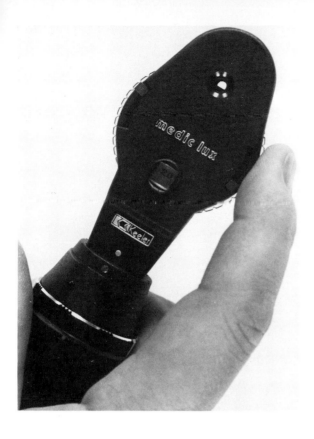

Figure 2.
Position of hand on
ophthalmoscope.

For focusing, the head of the direct ophthalmoscope contains a series of convex and concave lenses housed in a rotary disc. The convex or plus (+) lenses customarily are indicated by black numbers; the concave or minus (−) power lenses, by red numbers. The power of the lenses provided usually ranges from zero (plano) to plus and minus 15 or 20 diopters; in some instruments accessory lenses are included to provide as much as 40 diopters of lens power. To bring the image into focus, the examiner need only rotate the disc or 'dial in' sufficient power. The power or 'number' of the lens required will vary with the refractive state of both the examiner's eye and the patient's eye. If the examiner's refractive error is corrected with eye glasses, only the patient's refractive error need be neutralized or compensated for with the lenses. If the patient is very myopic and the examiner is having difficulty focusing on the retina, it may be helpful if the patient also puts on his glasses.

EXAMINATION TECHNIQUE

The instrument should be held securely, with the hand placed sufficiently far up on the barrel so that the forefinger can reach the rotary lens disc comfortably at all times (Fig. 2). This enables the examiner to change the dioptric power as needed throughout the examination.

The examiner uses his right hand and his right eye to examine the patient's right eye, his left hand and left eye to examine the patient's left eye.

3

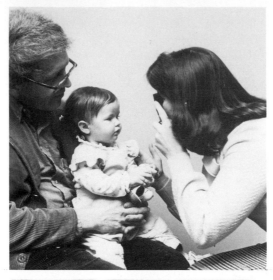

Figure 3.
Examination in the upright sitting position. Moving in slowly, one can often examine the optic fundus without upsetting or restraining child.

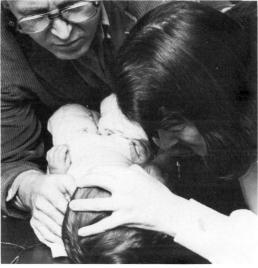

Figure 4.
Examination of infant lying on a flat surface. Child can be adequately and safely restrained by parent.

Both the examiner and patient must be positioned comfortably. With a little wooing, most children can be examined in the upright sitting position (Fig. 3). Infants often are better examined lying on a flat surface (Fig. 4) or cradled in the parent's arms. Examination also can be done well with the infant lying in the parent's lap with the baby's head resting on the knees and with his legs straddling the waist. By raising the baby's arms beside his head, the parent can restrain the infant securely but gently, while the examiner, sitting knee-to-knee with the parent, looks down over the top of the infant's head. It is also helpful if the infant sucks on a pacifier or bottle during the procedure.

Patience and a non-threatening approach are crucial to the successful examination of children. In the beginning it is important to touch the child as little as possible. In many cases, however, it becomes necessary to hold open the lids manually, or to restrain the child; this must be done gently, preferably by a member of the family or by an attendant

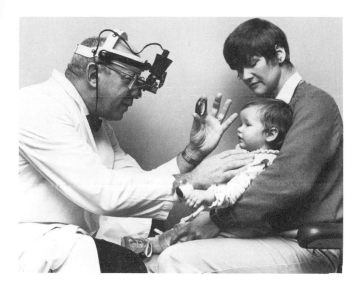

Figure 5.
Indirect
ophthalmoscopy.
Head lamp and
hand-held
condensing lens
are used to
visualize the optic
fundus.

experienced in handling apprehensive youngsters. The frightful practice of strapping down a child is to be avoided. Talking to the child, humming or playing soft music during the procedure may also help to calm the child.

Visualization of the inner eye can be augmented or facilitated by dilating the pupils with mydriatic eyedrops.

Systematic ophthalmoscopy begins with examination of the outer eye and assessment of the clarity of the 'red reflex' (the reddish-orange glow of light reflected from the retina through the optical media). A high plus lens (10 to 15 diopters) is used, with the instrument held 12 inches or so from the eye. Any opacity such as a cataract or vitreous floater will cast a dark shadow in the reflex. The reflex also may appear dark if the patient has a high refractive error.

The examiner then progressively moves closer to the eye, simultaneously reducing the plus power in the instrument by rotating the lens disc counterclockwise (toward the minus side), gradually focusing more deeply into the eye until the structures of the fundus come into clear view.

It is customary to examine the optic disc first; then each of the four quadrants of the fundus, following the major vessel branches as far as possible; and finally the macula. The disc is best seen by having the patient look forward, while the examiner directs the light just nasal to the patient's line of gaze. If one is 'lost' in the fundus, the disc can be located by tracing the major vessels back to their origin. The more peripheral regions can be brought into view by having the patient look as far as possible in the direction of the intended examination, *i.e.* up and to the right for examination of the right-upper temporal quadrant, down and to the left for examination of the left-inferior temporal quadrant, and so forth. The macula is brought into view by asking the patient to look directly into the examiner's light. Examination of the far periphery requires full pupillary dilatation and use of the indirect ophthalmoscope; skilful use of this instrument requires considerable practice and is often left to the ophthalmologist (Fig. 5).

THE NORMAL FUNDUS

The area of the fundus occupied by the ophthalmoscopically visible intra-ocular portion of the optic nerve is referred to as the disc. Anatomically it is referred to as the nervehead or papilla. It is composed of approximately 1 million nerve fibers converging from the retina to course through the optic nerve, chiasm and tracts to the lateral geniculate body. The structure is round to slightly oval, averaging 1.5 to 1.7mm, with its long axis vertical. It is somewhat nasal to the center of the globe. Often the nasal portion is fuller or more 'heaped up' than the temporal, owing to the greater number of nerve fibers coming into the nasal sector. The margins should be well defined. Normally the color is orange, ranging from yellow to pink. There is usually a paler central or paracentral depression referred to as the cup, occupying 30 per cent or less of the disc area. The major retinal vessels emerge from and converge into the cup area.

As the axons turn to course posteriorly into the nerve trunk, they traverse a sieve-like portion of the sclera, referred to as the cribiform plate. On ophthalmoscopic examination, grayish markings of this structure can often be visualized in the depth of the cup.

The central retinal artery emerging from the disc bifurcates into superior and inferior segments, each of which then divides into temporal and nasal branches that supply the four retinal quadrants. The vessels continue to branch further as they extend peripherally, curving gently in their course. On ophthalmoscopic examination the arteries (or, more correctly, arter-ioles) appear bright red with a lighter central stripe of reflected light.

The retinal veins converging into the disc follow a similar pattern of gently curving bifurcations, closely approximating those of the arterioles. Compared to the arterioles, the veins appear darker in color; they are also wider, having a ratio of 3:2 in diameter, and are somewhat more tortuous. Pulsation of the central retinal vein at the disc often can be seen as a normal finding.

The general background appearance of the fundus varies with the

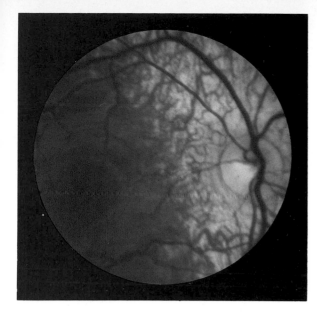

Figure A.
The normal fundus.
Landmarks are indicated in
the accompanying line
drawing.

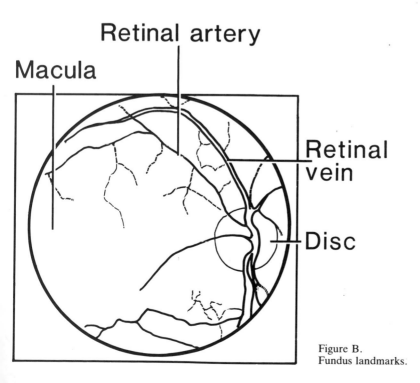

Retinal artery

Macula

Retinal
vein

Disc

Figure B.
Fundus landmarks.

chorioretinal pigmentation. In deeply pigmented individuals the fundus has a uniform to somewhat mottled dark reddish, brick or slate color. In lightly pigmented individuals the fundus appears a paler yellowish-orange to light red, and the underlying choroidal vessels and sclera can be seen more clearly as interlacing broad ribbons of reddish-orange hue. The intervening areas of sclera visible to ophthalmoscopic examination appear pale yellow to white. Peripherally, the swirling orange pattern of large collecting veins, the vortex veins, may be seen.

The central area of the fundus, ophthalmoscopically and functionally, is the macula or foveal region. This is the highly specialized area of the retina that serves as the visual center of the eye, providing man's best visual acuity. The macula encompasses an area somewhat larger than the disc, approximately two disc diameters temporal to the disc. Owing to its highly specialized histological features, the macula is a slightly elevated mound with a shallow depression at its center. On ophthalmoscopic examination it generally appears somewhat darker than the rest of the fundus; in many individuals the mound is highlighted by soft light reflexes or demarcated by a narrow ring of light, and the central pit is marked by a bright focal light reflex or yellowish spot. The retinal vessels arch above and below the macula but do not extend directly into the macula, although a cilioretinal vessel coursing from the disc to the macula is present in some individuals.

With regard to general localization ophthalmoscopically, the area in and immediately around the macula is also referred to as the posterior pole. The area around the disc is called the peripapillary area; the intermediate zone is called the mid-periphery; and the region beyond is the far-periphery.

THE ABNORMAL FUNDUS

PAPILLEDEMA

Papilledema is characterized by various degrees of congestion, swelling and elevation of the nervehead; obliteration of the disc cup; edematous blurring of the disc margins; dilatation and tortuosity of the retinal veins; loss of spontaneous venous pulsation; and hemorrhages and exudates on and around the disc (Fig. 1a,b,c). There also may be concentric wrinkling of the retina, and extension of the edema, hemorrhages and exudates into the macular area.

Papilledema or 'choked disc' is of primary clinical importance as a cardinal sign of increased intracranial pressure. Swelling of the disc may occur, however, with a variety of other neurological processes and systemic diseases, and with a number of ocular and orbital conditions of diverse etiology (Fig. 1d).

The probable sequence of events producing papilledema in patients with increased intracranial pressure is as follows: elevation of intracranial subarachnoid cerebrospinal fluid pressure; elevation of cerebrospinal fluid pressure in the sheath of the optic nerve; elevation of tissue pressure in the optic nerve; stasis of axoplasmic flow; and swelling of the nerve fibers in the optic nervehead. The axon swelling then produces secondary vascular changes and the characteristic ophthalmoscopic signs of venous stasis.

In children, papilledema most often is associated with hydrocephalus, intracranial tumor, intracranial hemorrhage, or the cerebral edema of trauma, meningo-encephalitis or toxic encephalopathy. It should be noted, however, that in the infant or very young child with increased intracranial pressure, papilledema may not develop owing to distensibility of the skull and spreading of the cranial sutures.

As a rule, papilledema will resolve when the elevated intracranial pressure is alleviated, and the discs may return to a normal or nearly normal appearance within six to eight weeks. However, longstanding papilledema may lead to postpapilledema optic atrophy with attendant loss of vision and visual field.

To be differentiated from true papilledema are certain structural changes of the disc ('pseudopapilledema', 'pseudoneuritis', drusen and medullated fibers) that can mimic the appearance of disc swelling.

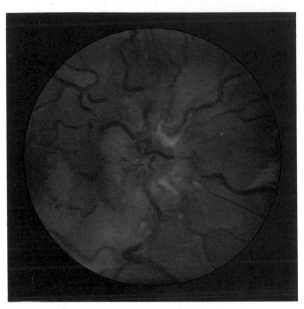

Figure 1a
Papilledema of increased intracranial pressure
There is hyperemia and swelling of nervehead, edema of retina, congestion and tortuosity of veins. Child had hydrocephalus.

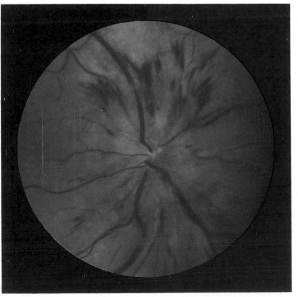

Figure 1b
Acute papilledema
In this patient with 'choked disc' of increased intracranial pressure, retinal hemorrhages are a prominent feature.

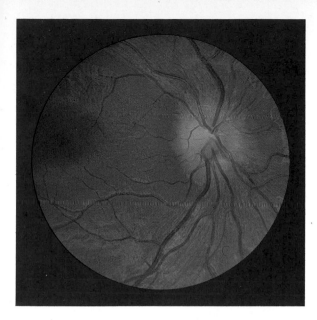

Figure 1c
Low-grade papilledema
Disc changes are minimal
in this child with increased
intracranial pressure
secondary to an infiltrative
tumor around aqueduct of
Sylvius. Child presented
with ataxia.

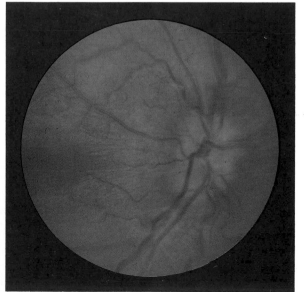

Figure 1d
Disc edema
Swelling of disc in this child
was due to histiocytosis
(Hand-Schueller-Christian
disease).

2 OPTIC NEURITIS

Optic neuritis exists when there is active inflammation, degeneration or demyelinization of the optic nerve with attendant impairment of visual function. When the anterior portion of the nerve is involved, producing ophthalmoscopically visible disc changes, the term *papillitis* is applied; this is characterized by edema or swelling of the nervehead (Fig. 2a,b), often with hemorrhages and exudates. When there is nervehead and retinal involvement, the term optic *neuroretinitis* can be used. When the more posterior intra-orbital, intracanalicular or intracranial portion of the nerve is involved, producing no ophthalmoscopically visible nervehead changes, the term *retrobulbar neuritis* is applied. The condition may be unilateral or bilateral.

Optic neuritis generally is an acute process, accompanied by visual symptoms that commence abruptly and progress rapidly; the involved eye may become blind or nearly blind in a matter of hours or days, although often vision loss is less profound or in some cases even minimal. A variety of visual-field defects occur, of which central and centrocecal scotomas are most common. There is usually an attendant afferent pupillary defect. There may be pain on movement of the eye or on palpation of the eyes; discomfort or headache may precede or accompany the visual symptoms.

Optic neuritis rarely occurs in childhood as an isolated entity; it is usually a manifestation of more widespread neurological or systemic disease. It may occur with demyelinating disease such as disseminated sclerosis, Devic's neuromyelitis optica or Schilder's disease (adrenoleukodystrophy). It may also occur in association with infectious or para-infectious processes, often as a complication of bacterial or viral meningitis, or as a complication of encephalomyelitis, particularly following an exanthem, or even an immunization. Certain toxins should also be considered in the etiology of optic neuritis in children—for example, it may develop with lead poisoning, as a complication of long-term, high-dose chloramphenicol therapy, with certain antimetabolites, or as the result of the use of illicit drugs.

The prognosis in optic neuritis varies with the etiology. In many cases there is recovery, with improvement in vision; in other cases there is permanent visual impairment and some degree of optic atrophy.

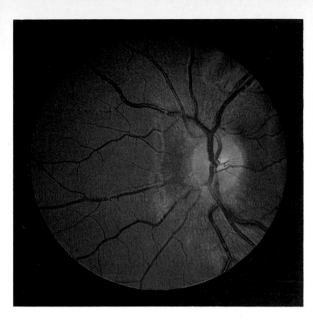

Figure 2a
Optic neuritis, acute
Note nerve-fiber layer edema. This 10-year-old patient presented with sudden loss of vision. She subsequently developed transverse myelitis, suggesting Devic's neuromyelitis optica.

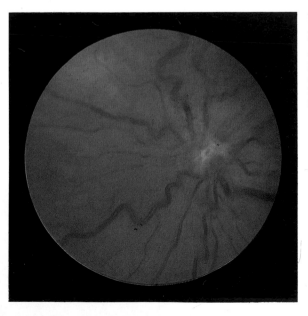

Figure 2b
Acute papillitis
This child developed acute optic neuritis consequent to long-term high-dose chloramphenicol treatment for cystic fibrosis. There is marked swelling of disc.

3 OPTIC ATROPHY

The term optic atrophy denotes degeneration of optic-nerve fibers with attendant impairment of function. The ophthalmoscopic signs are pallor and decreased vascularity of the disc, and loss of nervehead tissue, sometimes with enlargement of the optic cup (Fig. 3a,b,c,d). Clinical signs of impaired function vary with the nature and site of the primary lesion or disease process, and with the extent and severity of the damage; there may be localized visual-field defects, reduction or loss of central visual acuity, and signs of afferent (conduction) pupillary dysfunction.

Optic atrophy may result from disease within the eye or from disease affecting the intra-orbital, intracanalicular or intracranial portion of the anterior visual pathways. The causes are protean, including inflammatory processes, degenerative disorders, neoplastic disease, vascular disorders, trauma and toxic insults. Delineation of the etiology often requires extensive investigation, including neuroradiological, metabolic and genetic studies. However, the following generalizations may be of some practical clinical value in assessing children with optic atrophy.

Many children with optic atrophy have a readily identifiable, reasonable explanation for the atrophy. The problem often is long-standing and the course relatively stable. In this group are children with a well-documented past history of hypoxia or meningo-encephalitis and those with hydrocephalus, micrencephaly or craniosynostosis, or previous cranial trauma. There often is attendant developmental delay, a motor handicap, or seizure disorder. These children present little problem with regard to diagnosis, although documented progressive changes in the disc would warrant further investigation.

The previously normal child who develops progressive optic atrophy presents an entirely different diagnostic problem, and requires aggressive investigation for progressive neurological or systemic disease, intra-orbital or intracranial tumor. Craniopharyngioma, optic glioma and hydrocephalus are particularly frequent causes. A number of heredodegenerative optic atrophies that present in childhood also must be considered; diagnosis is based on careful family study and the clinical profile. In addition, glaucoma (increased intra-ocular pressure) must be ruled out in children with optic atrophy, particularly when there is enlargement or excavation of the optic cup.

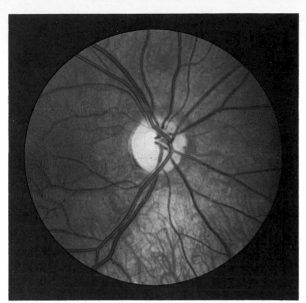

Figure 3a
Optic atrophy
This is the classical picture
of advanced optic atrophy.
Note pallor and decreased
vascularity of disc, and loss
of nervehead substance.

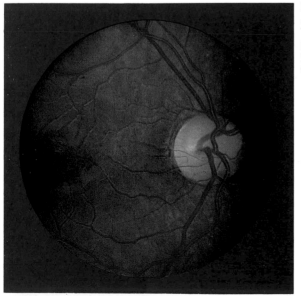

Figure 3b
Moderate optic atrophy
There is mild generalized
pallor of disc in this five
year-old child with
craniopharyngioma.

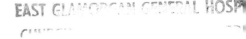

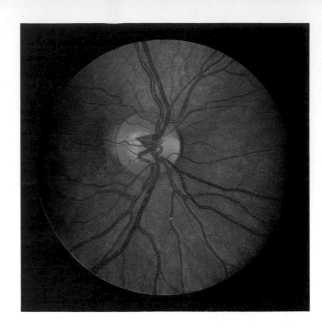

Figure 3c
Sector optic atrophy
In this child sector atrophy can be detected in temporal and nasal portions of disc as an early sign of brain tumor (craniopharyngioma).

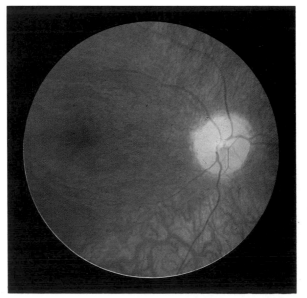

Figure 3d
Optic atrophy
Optic atrophy in this child is secondary to diffuse progressive nervous-system degeneration (lipofuscinosis). Note arteriolar attenuation.

OPTIC-CUP ENLARGEMENT

A large or enlarged optic cup may occur as a normal developmental variant or as the result of disease.

In the absence of disease, the developmentally large cup, though broad and deep, tends to be relatively round or only slightly oval, and is surrounded by a rim of healthy nervehead tissue (Fig. 4a). In addition, within the spectrum of normal variation, the cup is usually equal or nearly equal in the two eyes. Genetic determination is a factor in cup size, and examination of other family members may be helpful in differential diagnosis.

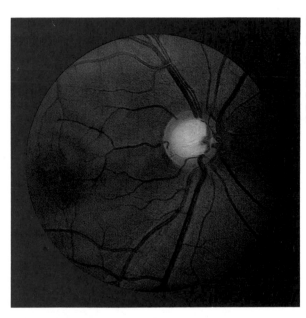

Figure 4a
Large disc cup
Vision and intra-ocular pressure were normal in this 10-year old boy with symmetrically large deep optic cups. Note rim of normal, pink nervehead tissue.

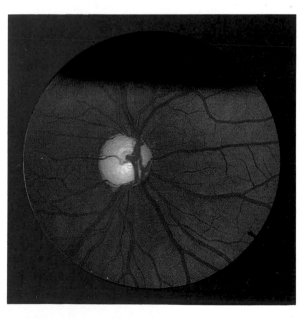

Figure 4b
Glaucomatous cupping
In this eight-year-old boy cup is enlarged and excavated, with pallor and atrophy of neuroretinal rim. Intra-ocular pressure was elevated abnormally and vision had been reduced to light perception. Fellow eye was normal.

To be differentiated from normal developmental variants are anomalies of the disc—colobomatous defects of the nervehead and optic-nerve hypoplasia, that may be characterized by the appearance of excavation.

Pathological enlargement and excavation of the cup, commonly referred to as 'cupping', is associated with glaucoma (Fig. 4b). In glaucoma the cup tends to show vertically oval or irregular enlargement, with pallor and atrophy of the neuroretinal rim, sometimes with 'notching' of the superior and inferior pole. The vessels also tend to become displaced nasally. In addition, significant difference between the cups of the two eyes is particularly suggestive of glaucoma. In infants and young children, other major signs of glaucoma are clouding (edema) of the cornea, photophobia and tearing, and progressive enlargement of the eye and cornea, referred to as buphthalmos. Ultimately there may be loss of vision.

In optic atrophy of other etiologies there may be some enlargement of the cup, but usually not the characteristic excavation and notching that occurs with the increased intra-ocular pressure of glaucoma.

OPTIC-NERVE PITS

Optic-nerve pits or 'holes' are considered to be minimal colobomatous defects. They appear as small round, oval, or slit-like craters or depressions, usually situated in the temporal portion of the disc (Fig. 5). There is often a diaphanous veil of grayish tissue filling-in or covering the defect. Optic-nerve pits may be associated with serous retinal detachment, and with vision and field defects that must be differentiated from those of progressive neurological disease.

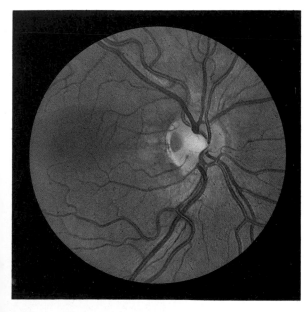

Figure 5
Optic pit
Note grayish oval defect in temporal portion of nervehead.

6 OPTIC-NERVE HYPOPLASIA

Optic-nerve hypoplasia is a developmental defect characterized by deficiency of optic-nerve fibers. It has been attributed to primary failure in the differentiation of retinal ganglion cells or their axons. However, it may result from prenatal degeneration of the ganglion-cell axons.

The defect may be unilateral or bilateral, mild to severe, with a broad spectrum of ophthalmoscopic findings and attendant clinical manifestations.

In typical cases the nervehead is small, occupying only a portion of the usual disc area, and leaving a pale or pigmented crescent or halo between the margin of the existent nervehead tissue and the margin of the pigmented retinal epithelium and choroid. This gives rise to the so-called 'double-ring' sign of optic-nerve hypoplasia. The nervehead tissue present usually is pale, although sometimes relatively pink. Paucity of tissue, however, is the principal diagnostic criterion (Fig. 6a,b,c,d). The major vessels generally are normal, although in some cases they are tortuous or attenuated. There is attendant hypoplasia of the macula; it appears flat, lacking its normal contours and light reflexes.

The attendant vision impairments range in severity from localized visual-field defects or minimal reduction in acuity to blindness of one or both eyes. In association with vision impairment there is often strabismus or nystagmus; abnormal eye movements or malalignment may be the presenting sign.

Optic-nerve hypoplasia may occur as an isolated defect in otherwise normal individuals, or in association with other abnormalities including anencephaly, hydranencephaly, hydrocephalus and meningo-encephalocele.

Hypoplasia of the optic nerves, chiasm and optic tracts may occur in association with absence of the septum pellucidum with a large chiasmatic cistern, an anomaly referred to as septo-optic dysplasia or deMorsier syndrome. There may be associated hypothalamic involvement, with endocrine disorders ranging from panhypopituitarism to isolated deficiency of growth hormone, hypothyroidism, diabetes insipidus or diabetes mellitus.

The exact cause of optic-nerve hypoplasia is unknown. It does not appear to be familial, although it has occurred in siblings. There is no chromosomal defect regularly associated with it. It may occur with somewhat increased frequency in infants of diabetic mothers.

To be differentiated from optic-nerve hypoplasia is optic-nerve aplasia. This is a rare anomaly in which there is absence of the optic nerve and of the retinal vessels. This condition presumably results from failure of the paraxial mesoderm to grow into the optic stalk before closure of the fetal fissure. Optic-nerve aplasia rarely occurs in otherwise normal individuals. It is usually associated with malformation of the globes or brain.

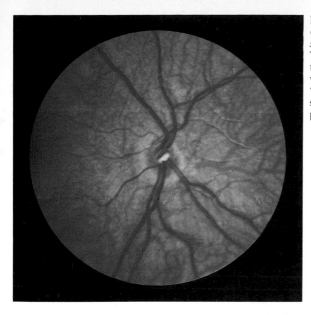

Figure 6a
Optic-nerve hypoplasia of severe degree
There is minimal nervehead tissue around central retinal vessels. Note pale halo or 'double-ring sign' encircling small donut of pink papillary tissue.

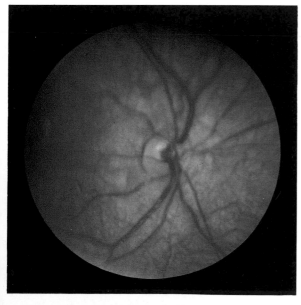

Figure 6b
Optic-nerve hypoplasia of moderate degree
Disc is just slightly smaller than normal, relatively pink, but flat and slightly deficient in nervehead tissue.

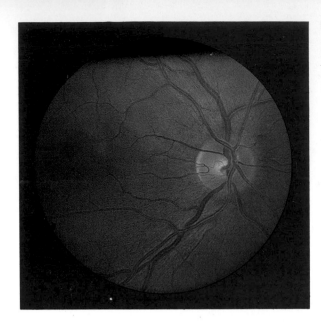

Figure 6c
Optic-nerve hypoplasia of minimal degree
Nervehead is small. There is only slight indication of a partial peripapillary ring.

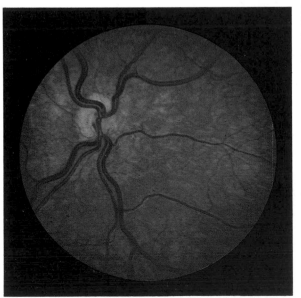

Figure 6d
Typical double-ring sign of optic-nerve hypoplasia
Double-ring sign in this infant is prominent.

TILTED DISC

Tilted optic disc is an anomaly in which one portion of the disc is displaced forward and appears elevated or 'full'; the opposite sector of the disc appears flat or recessed and often is bordered with a crescent or conus (Fig. 7). The disc may be tilted in any direction. The condition usually is bilateral. This anomaly is thought to be related to malclosure of the embryonic fissure. In conjunction with tilted disc there may be myopia and astigmatism, and vision and visual-field defects. The field defects often are bitemporal or altitudinal, and must be differentiated from those of acquired or progressive disease. In addition, the appearance of a tilted disc may mimic that of papilledema, as the margin of the elevated segment of the disc may appear 'blurred' on ophthalmoscopic examination.

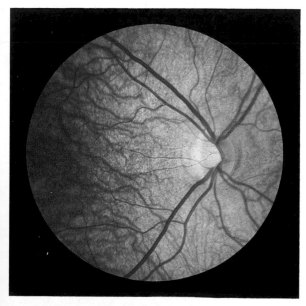

Figure 7
Tilted disc
Disc appears to be 'facing' macula; nasal portion of nervehead is prominent and displaced forward; the temporal portion of nervehead appears recessed and foreshortened; vessels appear to emerge from beneath temporal rim; and there is a pale crescent along temporal margin of disc.

Optic-disc drusen are globular, acellular bodies composed of concentric lamellae of hyalin material. They may be buried within the optic nervehead, producing smooth or irregular elevation of the disc that can be confused with papilledema (Fig. 8). Alternatively, the drusen may be partially or completely exposed, appearing as refractile bodies resembling tapioca pearls at the surface of the disc. The more superficial disc drusen often can be made to glow when transilluminated with oblique light. Fluorescein angiography, ultrasonography and computed axial tomography of the optic nerve also are useful in documenting the presence of intrapapillary drusen.

In some instances disc drusen are associated with nerve-fiber bundle or sector visual-field defects, enlargement of the blind spot, decreased visual acuity, and even with small spontaneous nerve fiber-layer hemorrhages adjacent to the disc.

The etiology of optic-disc drusen is unclear. They may occur as an autosomal dominant condition; examination of other family members may be helpful in making the diagnosis. Giant drusen of the disc have been associated with tuberous sclerosis of Bourneville.

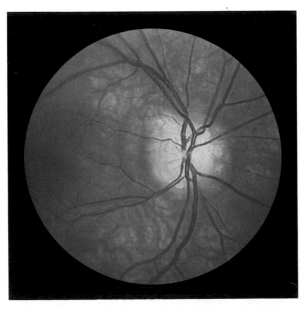

Figure 8
Optic-disc drusen
Note nodular elevation of nervehead and irregularity of disc margins due to hyalin bodies. Child was referred for evaluation of suspected papilledema; the clinical picture is that of pseudopapilledema.

PERSISTENT BERGMEISTER PAPILLA— EPIPAPILLARY MEMBRANE

Persistence of Bergmeister's papilla, often taking the form of an epipapillary membrane or glial tuft protruding from the disc, is a common developmental remnant.

Embryologically, as nerve fibers grow into the primitive epithelial papilla to form the optic nerve, a nidus of neuro-ectodermal cells becomes sequestered from the rest of the inner layer of the optic cup. At about the end of the fourth gestational month these cells multiply and form a glial sheath that extends around the hyaloid artery. During the seventh

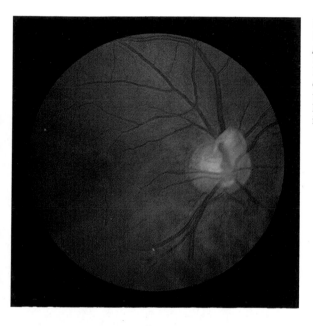

Figure 9a
Persistent Bergmeister papilla
Incomplete regression of Bergmeister's papilla in this child has left translucent tissue over disc with a cyst-like structure protruding into vitreous.

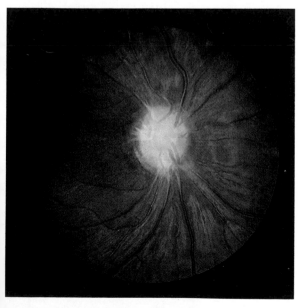

Figure 9b
Glial papillary veil
Persistent glial tissue over disc, as shown in this otherwise normal child, should not be confused with papilledema or papillitis. This is a developmental variant.

gestational month this tissue begins to atrophy. Incomplete regression may leave varying amounts of glial tissue. Ophthalmoscopically the appearance ranges from barely detectable glial tufts to conspicuous whitish veils over the disc, or globular or finger-like structures protruding into the vitreous (Fig. 9a,b). As a rule these developmental remnants do not affect visual function. These common developmental variants generally are easily recognized and should not be confused with inflammatory, hamartomatous or neoplastic conditions. The veils also must be differentiated from the disc changes of papilledema or papillitis.

PERSISTENT HYPERPLASTIC PRIMARY VITREOUS (PHPV)

Remnants of the vascular and fibrous elements of the primary vitreous may persist to varying degrees anywhere from the disc to the posterior surface of the lens, and in some individuals there is associated fibroblastic hyperplasia. This condition in its various forms is referred to as persistent hyperplastic primary vitreous or PHPV (Fig. 10a,b).

In full-blown or classical PHPV there is a retrolental mass or opacity, giving rise to a white reflex in the pupil. There is often prominence of the ciliary processes. The affected eye usually is microphthalmic or somewhat

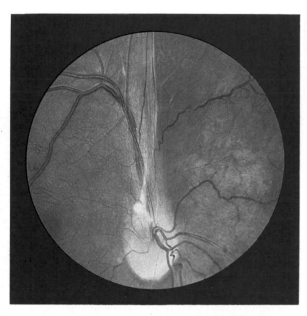

Figure 10a
Persistent hyperplastic primary vitreous
There is glial tissue extending superiorly from disc with associated traction on retina. Child subsequently developed a vitreous hemorrhage.

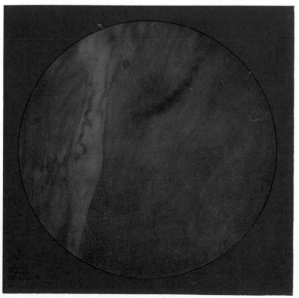

Figure 10b
PHPV
Note tube-like structure traversed by vessels lying anterior to retina. This is related to persistence of primary vitreous and hyaloid system.

smaller than normal. Associated complications include cataract, glaucoma, intra-ocular hemorrhage, retinal traction and detachment.

Lesser degrees of PHPV may be characterized by small remnants on the back surface of the lens. In other cases there is primarily involvement of the disc and retina. The ophthalmoscopic picture is often that of glial tissue over the disc. Fibroglial proliferation in the region of the disc may produce traction on the retina, leading to retinal fold or detachment.

In most cases PHPV is unilateral. Other ocular defects and systemic anomalies have been noted in some cases.

An unusual disc anomaly sometimes associated with PHPV, or possibly related developmentally to the whole spectrum of PHPV, is the so-called 'morning glory' disc anomaly. It may occur in association with other developmental defects including cleft palate, absence of the corpus callosum, sphenoidal encephalocele and renal abnormalities.

MYELINATED NERVE FIBERS

Whereas myelination of the optic-nerve fibers normally terminates at the level of the lamina cribosa, in some individuals myelination continues anterior to the lamina cribosa, resulting in ectopic medullation of the fibers of the optic nervehead and of the retina. On ophthalmoscopic examination, this area appears as a white or grayish-white patch, having a striated or feathered edge (Fig. 11).

There may be a relative or absolute visual-field defect corresponding to the area of ectopic medullation, or associated refractive error (myopia), strabismus or ambylopia. Otherwise, the eye usually is normal, although a variety of defects, including coloboma and cranial anomalies, has been reported in association with ectopic medullation. Ectopic medullation is also said to occur with increased frequency in von Recklinghausen neurofibromatosis.

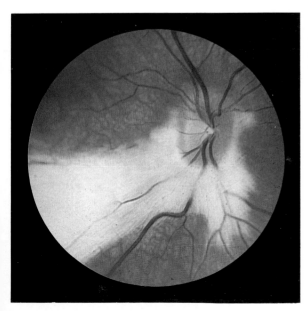

Figure 11
Medullated nerve fibers
This 'painted-on' brush-stroke appearance is characteristic of ectopic myelination of retinal-nerve fibers.

When the retinal-pigment epithelium or choroid fails to abut the margin of the disc, a peripapillary crescent may be seen (Fig. 12). This is a common developmental anomaly; congenital crescents are located most frequently on the temporal side of the disc and are often demarcated by extra pigmentation. They also occur in some individuals with myopia.

Developmental crescents usually are well defined and should not be confused with inflammatory or degenerative conditions.

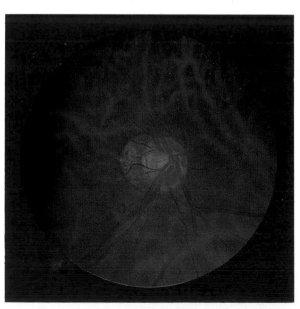

Figure 12
Peripapillary crescent
In this darkly pigmented child retinal-pigment epithelium falls short of disc margin, leaving a peripapillary choroidal crescent.

COLOBOMATA

The term coloboma describes a defect (gap, notch, fissure, hole) in which tissue or a portion of a tissue or structure is lacking. The principal types of ocular colobomata are (1) chorioretinal or fundus coloboma, with or without iris, ciliary body or optic-nerve involvement; and (2) isolated optic-nerve coloboma.

The typical fundus coloboma arises from malclosure of the embryonic fissure; this results in a defect in the retina, retinal-pigment epithelium and choroid, baring the sclera. The usual appearance is that of a well-circumscribed, wedge-shaped white area (exposed sclera) extending inferonasally below the disc, sometimes involving or engulfing the disc (Fig. 13a,b). In extreme cases there is cyst formation or ectasia in the area of the cleft. Alternatively, chorioretinal colobomata may be small focal defects appearing as single or multiple punched-out lesions or pigmentation in the line of the embryonic fissure (Fig. 13c,d). The defect may be unilateral or bilateral.

As a rule, there is a visual-field defect corresponding to the area of the chorioretinal defect. Visual acuity may be impaired, particularly if the optic nerve or macula is involved. The visual-field defects of this congenital anomaly must be differentiated from those of progressive disease.

Chorioretinal colobomata may occur unassociated with other abnormalities, as a sporadic defect or inherited as a dominant or recessive condition, or in association with other anomalies such as microphthalmia, cyclopia or anencephaly. They may occur in the syndromes of Patau (trisomy 13) or Edward (trisomy 18), with significant CNS abnormalties.

Isolated coloboma of the optic nerve, without the typical chorioretinal defect, may occur as a rare anomaly. In this condition the disc appears larger than normal, there is excavation and distortion of the disc, sometimes with a glial veil over the crater, and the blood vessels appear to traverse the border of the defect. There may be associated impairment of vision or field, but this is variable. This anomaly may be associated with trans-sphenoidal encephalocele, as well as with other system anomalies such as cardiac defects and a number of ocular abnormalities including posterior embryotoxon and posterior lenticonus. It may be familial.

A disc anomaly that may be related to coloboma of the optic disc is the 'morning glory' disc anomaly. In this condition the disc appears large with a funnel-shaped excavation and an annulus of elevated peripapillary tissue, sometimes pigmented. In some cases vision is subnormal. A variety of developmental abnormalities, including cleft lip and palate, agenesis of the corpus callosum and sphenoidal encephalocele, have been reported in association with the disc anomaly.

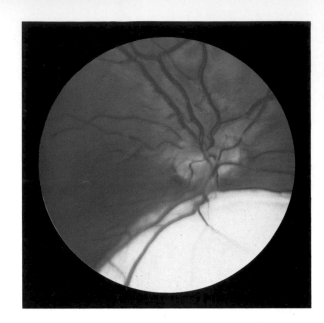

Figure 13a
Typical fundus coloboma
A well-demarcated
chorioretinal defect extends
inferonasally below disc. A
wedge-shaped area of sclera
is exposed.

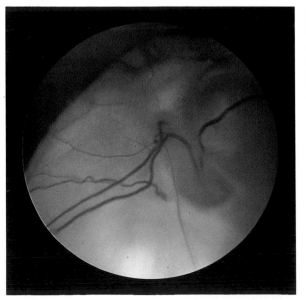

Figure 13b
Coloboma involving disc
This fundus coloboma
extends proximally,
engulfing disc. There is
marked distortion of disc
and vessels, and sclera is
ectatic.

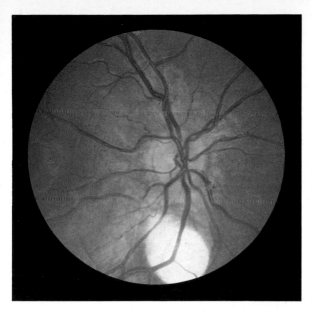

Figure 13c
*Focal chorioretinal
coloboma*
There is a discrete defect
inferior to disc; retinal
vessels traverse exposed
sclera.

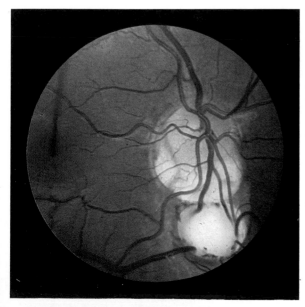

Figure 13d
*Fundus coloboma involving
disc*
In this child malclosure of
the embryonic fissure has
resulted in array of
contiguous defects. Note (1)
crescent-shaped defect
involving lower pole of disc;
(2) adjacent cavernous or
cyst-like defect with vessels
'climbing' rim; and (3)
sector of hypopigmentation
around defects and disc.

In clinical practice the term chorioretinitis is used in a broad sense to describe a variety of inflammatory changes of the choroid and retina. Pathologically, inflammation may arise primarily in the retina or in the choroid; the inflammation may be confined to these tissues, or the fundus changes may be just one facet of more extensive ocular inflammation.*

The causes are protean, and include both infectious and non-infectious processes. The clinical signs vary somewhat with the etiology, but certain generalizations can be made. As a rule, the acute phase is marked by cellular reaction with varying degrees of edema, exudation and hemorrhage; the involved areas of the fundus may appear hazy, gray or yellowish, there may be vascular sheathing, and the vitreous may appear cloudy owing to out-pouring of inflammatory cells (Fig. 14a,b). The process often results in necrosis and destruction of choroidal and retinal tissue, with dispersion and aggregation of pigment. In many cases the end result is permanent chorioretinal scarring—depending on the etiology and extent of the process, the ophthalmoscopic signs may vary from pigmentary mottling to discrete focal areas of chorioretinal atrophy appearing as white patches of exposed sclera, often well demarcated by dense clumps of pigmentation (Fig. 14c,d). There also may be gliotic veils or dense fibrotic membranes, retinal folds or detachment (Fig. 14e).

Whereas any number of infectious and non-infectious disease processes may be associated with chorioretinitis, those of special interest in pediatric practice are toxoplasmosis, cytomegalovirus disease and herpes virus infection, rubella, syphilis, tuberculosis and sarcoidosis, and toxocariasis.

The retinochoroiditis of congenital toxoplasmosis is usually characterized by focal atrophic and pigmented scars (Fig. 14f); large destructive lesions of the macular region are common. Rarely are there signs of active retinochoroiditis at birth. Active recurrences of the retinochoroiditis of toxoplasmosis may occur at any time in life, often resulting in satellite lesions adjacent to old scars. Detection of fundus lesions suggesting toxoplasmosis can be of diagnostic importance in the evaluation of an infant with signs of congenital infection syndrome, or in a child with developmental delay, retardation, microcephaly, intracranial calcifications or a seizure disorder.

Congenital cytomegalovirus infection and *Herpes simplex* infection acquired at birth may be seen as active chorioretinal inflammation in the infant, frequently accompanying signs of systemic infection or encephalitis. Vitreous haze, retinal edema and hemorrhages are common in the active phase; varying degrees of chorioretinal atrophy and pigmentation may follow. The chorioretinitis of *Herpes simplex* and cytomegalovirus may also

---

*It is common to classify ocular inflammation on the basis of the parts of the eye affected. Thus, inflammation of any part of the uveal tract generally can be referred to as uveitis, or more specifically as iritis, cyclitis, or choroiditis; it can be described as anterior or posterior uveitis depending on which segment is predominantly affected, or as panuveitis if all segments are involved. In many cases of uveitis there is inflammatory involvement of the contiguous retina, and the descriptive term chorioretinitis is applied. Similarly, inflammation arising in the retina may involve the underlying choroid; some prefer the term retinochoroiditis to make this distinction. Inflammation can be confined to the retina, and may be referred to as retinitis or as retinal vasculitis.

Visual symptoms vary considerably with the etiology and severity of the inflammatory process.

be seen as later-onset acquired disease, particularly as opportunistic infection in children on immunosuppressive therapy (Fig. 14g).

The fundus changes of congenital rubella are those of a pigmentary retinopathy, commonly of the 'salt and pepper' type, and are best described separately (see p. 41).

Congenital syphilis is relatively rare today, but may be seen as active choroiditis in the infant, or as secondary pigmentary changes detected later.

In sarcoidosis, retinal vascular signs are prominent. Perivenous infiltrates are common. There may be denser white inflammatory accumulations along retinal vessels resembling candle-wax drippings (Fig. 14h,i). Retinal edema, scattered exudates and hemorrhages also are common findings.

Tuberculous lesions in children are rarely seen, but miliary lesions of the choroid may develop in some children with generalized miliary tuberculosis and tuberculous meningitis. Clinically, these appear as ill-defined pale yellow, rounded lesions.

The fundus lesion of *Toxocara canis* usually is a unilateral focal lesion. On ophthalmoscopic examination it appears as an elevated white or grayish mass (Fig. 14j), most commonly located posteriorly in the macular region but sometimes situated peripherally along the ora serata, often with a transvitreal band. The vitreous may be hazy. The mass may give rise to the so-called cat's eye reflex or leukocoria—an opalescent reflection or white spot seen through the pupil.

As indicated by these few examples, in many patients with fundus signs of inflammatory disease, the clinical picture gives a clue to the etiology. It should be noted, however, that in many cases the signs are non-specific, and frequently the etiological agent cannot be identified, even after extensive investigation.

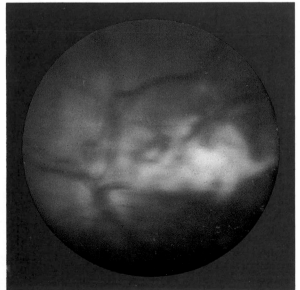

Figure 14a
Acute chorioretinitis
Acute inflammatory process is marked by exudation and edema, with haziness of fundus detail.

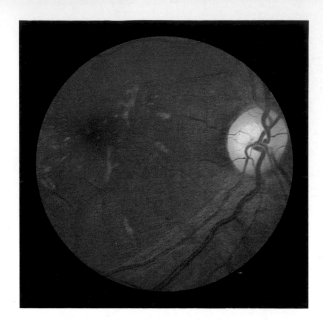

Figure 14b
Acute retinitis
Note retinal edema and exudation. Child presented with acute encephalitis, thought to be viral.

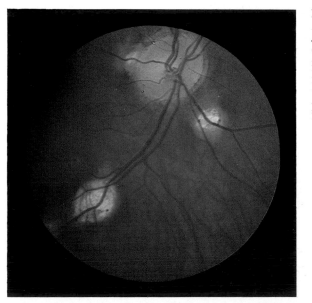

Figure 14c
Focal atrophic chorioretinal scars
Chorioretinitis often results in 'punched-out' atrophic lesions such as these. Child had familial chronic granulomatous disease and suffered multiple bouts of bacterial infection.

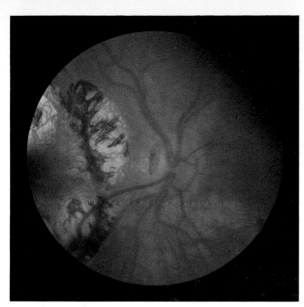

Figure 14d
Typical chorioretinal scar
Large areas of chorioretinal atrophy demarcated by dense pigmentation are common end-result of destructive inflammatory process in many patients with chorioretinitis.

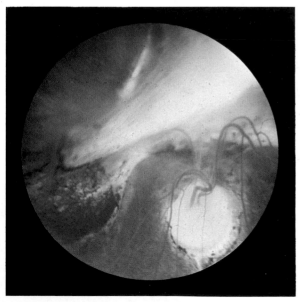

Figure 14e
Extensive chorioretinal scarring
Note chorioretinal atrophy, dense pigmentation, gliosis, retinal-vessel distortion and optic atrophy, all postinflammatory.

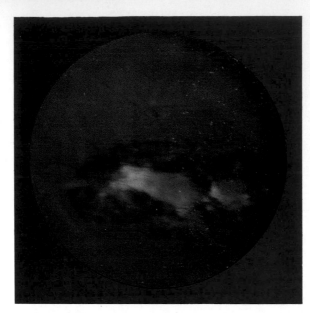

Figure 14f
Toxoplasmic chorioretinal scar
Large atrophic and pigmented scar near macula in this young girl with toxoplasmosis is typical of destructive lesions that so often occur in this disease. Satellite lesions are common.

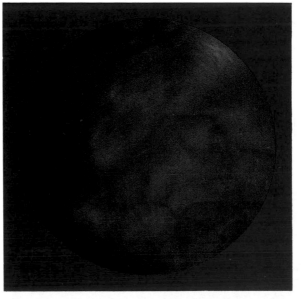

Figure 14g
Cytomegalovirus chorioretinitis
There is widespread edema and exudation of acute inflammation. This black child was on immunosuppressive drugs following kidney transplant.

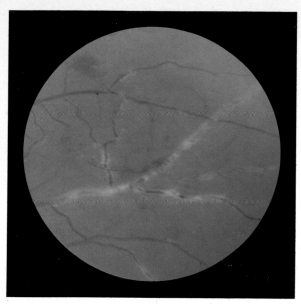

Figure 14h
Sarcoid retinitis
Perivascular exudates, likened to candle-wax drippings, retinal edema and scattered retinal hemorrhages are prominent features in this young boy with sarcoidosis.

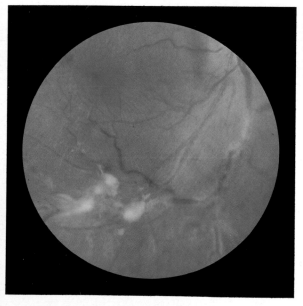

Figure 14i
Sarcoid retinitis
Note haze of widespread edema, perivascular exudates, and retinal hemorrhages.

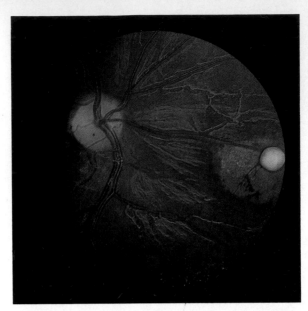

Figure 14j
Toxocara lesion
In this child with toxocariasis, there is elevated cystic lesion contiguous to a retinal vessel, in association with background pigmentary changes of fundus.

'SALT AND PEPPER' RETINOPATHY

'Salt and pepper' retinopathy is not a specific entity but rather a descriptive term applied to the retinal pigmentary changes seen in a number of diseases. The ophthalmoscopic picture is that of fine to coarse pigment stippling or mottling, alternating light and dark spots of pigment loss and pigment clumping.

A classic example is the retinopathy of congenital rubella (Fig. 15a,b). Typically, there is fine to coarse pigment clumping or mottling. The changes may be generalized, or predominantly central or peripheral, unilateral or bilateral. The retinopathy may occur as the sole ocular stigmata of the disease, or in association with other ocular changes of congenital rubella such as cataract, glaucoma or microphthalmos. The retinal changes usually are stationary from birth and rarely progressive, although a late complication characterized by sudden macular hemorrhage and vision impairment may occur years after birth.

The pigmentary changes of syphilitic retinitis may also be of the 'salt and pepper' type.

Certain acquired viral exanthems of childhood, particularly rubeolla, also may produce fine pigmentary changes.

To be differentiated from the retinal pigmentary changes of infectious diseases are the retinal signs of certain metabolic disorders. The retinopathy of cystinosis, for example, is characterized by fine to coarse pigment clumping in an otherwise hypopigmented fundus (Fig. 15c). The pigment stippling commonly appears first in the periphery but in time may be seen throughout the fundus. As a rule it is not associated with vision loss. Important to the diagnosis, of course, is the detection of cystine crystals in the cornea and conjunctiva.

Also to be differentiated are certain retinal degenerations that may present with fine to coarse pigment mottling—such changes may be associated with progressive systemic or neurological disease (see p. 44) (Fig. 15d). Associated signs, progression and deterioration of function are, of course, crucial in the differential diagnosis of such conditions.

Not to be confused with 'salt and pepper' retinopathy is the pigment stippling often seen as a normal developmental variation in some blond and red-headed children.

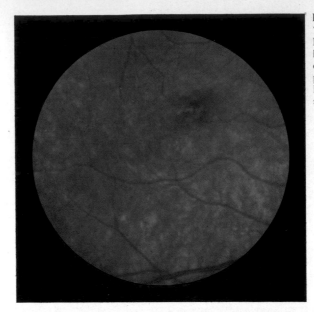

Figure 15a
'Salt and pepper' retinopathy
Note pattern of alternating light and dark spots, areas of depigmentation and pigment clumping. Child had congenital rubella syndrome.

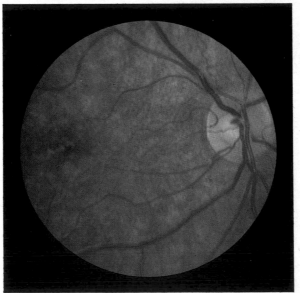

Figure 15b
Rubella retinopathy
In this child with congenital rubella there is coarse pigmentary mottling of posterior pole, and finer 'salt and pepper' stippling of other areas.

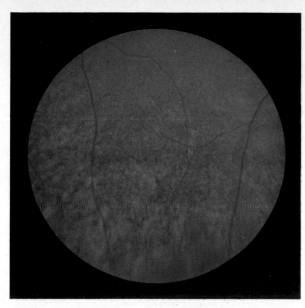

Figure 15c
Pigmentary retinopathy of cystinosis
The 'salt and pepper' pattern in this child is due to cystinosis. Retinopathy gave clue to diagnosis before corneal changes were documented by biomicroscopy.

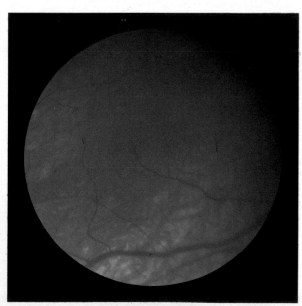

Figure 15d
Degeneration presenting with 'salt and pepper' changes
The coarse 'salt and pepper' type pigment changes in this infant with developmental delay, hypotonia and hepatomegaly, were the early manifestations of progressive neurological disease—Zellweger syndrome.

Pigmentary retinal degeneration is characterized by disorganization of the retinal pigmentary pattern, arteriolar attenuation, some degree of optic atrophy, and attendant impairment of visual function. Dispersion, migration and aggregation of retinal pigment produce a variety of ophthalmoscopically visible changes, ranging from fine granularity or coarse mottling to large focal aggregations of pigment with the configuration of bone spicules (Fig. 16a,b,c,d). The pigmentary changes usually appear first in the mid-periphery of the fundus, although in some cases the macula is affected first. Visual symptoms include impairment of dark adaptation, loss of peripheral field, often in the form of an expanding ring scotoma or concentric contraction of the visual field, and reduction of acuity. The ERG is reduced.

Pigmentary retinal degeneration may occur as an isolated ocular condition (classic 'retinitis pigmentosa'), as an inherited autosomal recessive, autosomal dominant, or sex-linked disorder; in association with other abnormalities as an expression of systemic, metabolic, or neurological disease; or as one feature of a multifaceted syndrome. It may be associated with polydactyly, obesity, hypogonadism and mental deficiency in the Laurence-Moon-Biedl syndrome; with abetalipoproteinemia and acanthocytosis as in the Bassen-Kornzweig syndrome; with progressive cerebellar ataxia and peripheral polyneuropathy in the Refsum syndrome; with hyperkinesia and mental retardation in Hallervorden-Spatz disease; or with progressive external ophthalmoplegia and heart block in the Kearns-Sayre syndrome. It can be a manifestation of generalized mucopolysaccharidosis, as in the syndromes of Hurler, Hunter, Scheie, and Sanfilippo, or as a manifestation of sphingolipidosis or lipofuscinosis, as in the syndromes of Batten-Mayou-Spielmeyer-Vogt or Jansky-Bielschowsky, to name just a few. Thus, in each case of pigmentary retinal degeneration consideration must be given to possible systemic, metabolic, neurological and genetic implications.

A type of pigmentary retinal degeneration or dystrophy of special importance in pediatrics is Leber's congenital amaurosis. In this condition the retinal changes are pleomorphic with varying degrees of pigment clumping and mottling. Severe vision impairment and an abnormal EEG are evident early.

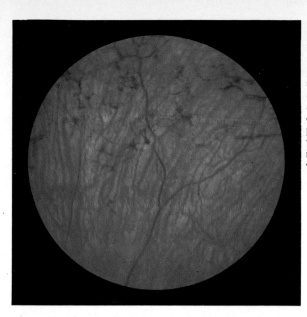

Figure 16a
Retinitis pigmentosa
These fundus changes are typical of retinitis pigmentosa. Note bone-spicule pigment aggregates, areas of pigment loss, and arteriolar attenuation. This otherwise healthy teenage patient suffered progressive vision loss beginning early in childhood. Her siblings were affected similarly.

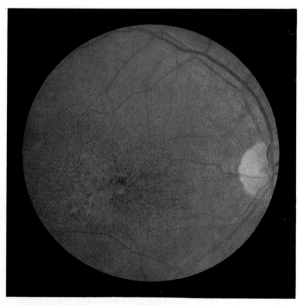

Figure 16b
Inverse retinitis pigmentosa
Subtle macular changes, disc pallor and decreasing visual acuity were first signs of retinitis pigmentosa in this otherwise normal eight-year-old female. Classic peripheral bone-spicule pigment aggregates developed in time.

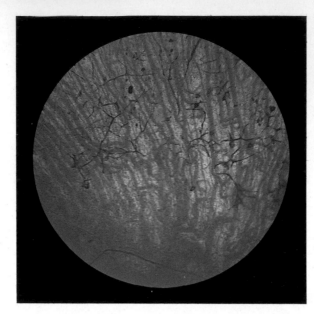

Figure 16c
*Pigmentary retinal
degeneration in ceroid
lipofuscinosis*
Retinitis pigmentosa-like
changes developed late in
childhood in this patient
with ceroid lipofuscinosis.
Child presented with
seizures and progressive loss
of abilities.

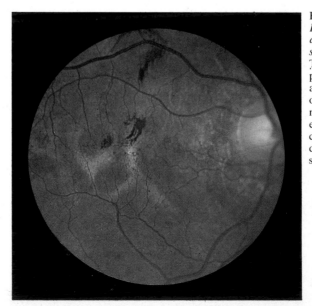

Figure 16d
*Pigmentary retinal
degeneration in a complex
syndrome*
These coarse retinal
pigmentary changes and
attendant vision loss
occurred in an adolescent
male with progressive
external ophthalmoplegia,
cerebellar ataxia and
dementia (PEO-plus
syndrome).

CHERRY-RED SPOT

The term 'cherry-red spot' describes the clinically detectable macular changes produced when transparency of the retinal ganglion cells is lost, usually as the result of edema or lipid accumulation. On ophthalmoscopic examination, the multilayer ganglion-cell ring of the macula appears hazy or thickened, and of grayish, white or yellow color. In contrast to this pale or creamy halo, the vascular blush of the underlying choroid at the center of the macula, an area essentially devoid of ganglion cells, appears bright or dark red (Fig. 17a,b).

In pediatric practice, the macular cherry-red spot is most important as a sign of the neuronal lipidoses. It characteristically occurs in Tay-Sachs disease (GM_2 type 1) and in the Sandoff variant (GM_2 type 2); it also occurs in some cases of generalized gangliosidoses (GM_1 type 1). Cherry-red-like macular changes also have been described in other sphingolipidoses, particularly the neuronopathic forms of Niemann-Pick disease (sphingo-myelin lipidosis) and Gaucher disease (glucosyl ceramide lipidosis), in some cases of metachromatic leukodystrophy (sulfatide lipidosis) and in certain mucolipidoses, namely Farber disease and Spranger disease. However, the clinically visible macular changes in these conditions tend to be less well defined or more subtle than those of the classic cherry-red spot of Tay-Sachs disease.

It is to be remembered that in many diseases a cherry-red spot is only the focal, ophthalmoscopically visible macular sign of more widespread retinal or generalized neuronal degeneration.

To be differentiated from the cherry-red spot of neurodegenerative disease is the cherry-red spot that may occur as the result of retinal ischemia, as with occlusion of the central retinal artery, or in association with the retinal edema of ocular contusion (Fig. 17c).

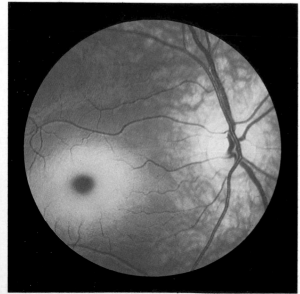

Figure 17a
Classical cherry-red spot
In this child with Tay-Sachs disease center of macula appears bright red in contrast to creamy pallor of macular ganglion-cell ring.

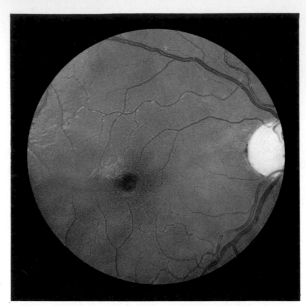

Figure 17b
Degenerated cherry-red spot
Over a period of years, the once brilliant cherry-red spot in this five-year-old child with Tay-Sachs disease degenerated, appearing 'burned-out'.

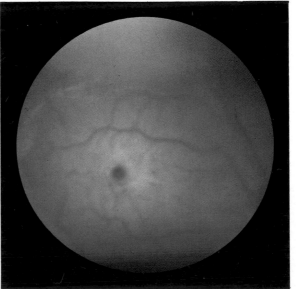

Figure 17c
Cherry-red spot of retinal ischemia
Unilateral cherry-red spot in this otherwise healthy 13-year-old girl was due to occlusion of central retinal artery. She suffered sudden loss of vision.

MACULAR DEGENERATION

There are many types of macular degeneration with variation in the pathological features and clinical manifestations. Of major importance in pediatric practice are the hereditary degenerations. Some occur alone, as genetically determined primary macular or retinal disorders, without associated systemic or neurological involvement. Others occur in association with systemic or neurological signs, as manifestations of more widespread metabolic or neurodegenerative disease.

Two important types of heredomacular degeneration unassociated with central nervous system involvement are Stargardt's juvenile macular degeneration and Best vitelliform macular degeneration.

As originally described by Stargardt, juvenile macular degeneration is characterized by slowly progressive macular deterioration and attendant vision loss, manifesting by age eight to 20 years (Fig. 18a). Initially, there may be only mild changes of the pigment epithelium, a beaten-copper or beaten-silver appearance, and later a picture of more advanced atrophy of the pigment epithelium in the macular region. In some cases there are white or yellowish spots around the macula or throughout the posterior fundus, and there may be mild pigmentary changes in the periphery; in such cases the term fundus flavimaculatus is used (Fig. 18b). The ERG and peripheral fields usually are normal. The condition is autosomal recessive.

In Best vitelliform macular degeneration the characteristic lesion is a yellow or orange discoid subretinal macular lesion, resembling the intact yolk of a fried egg. This usually is diagnosed between ages five and 15 years, and as a rule the vision is normal in the early stage. The fundus signs, however, are variable. In some cases the macular abnormality is subtle, with minimal pigmentary changes or alteration of the foveal appearance. Often there is progressive macular degeneration characterized by atrophy, pigmentation, fibrous scarring, and attendant vision impairment. As a rule the ERG is normal; the EOG is abnormal in affected individuals and in carriers. This degeneration usually is autosomal dominant.

Macular degenerations associated with central nervous system degeneration commonly are referred to as the cerebromacular degenerations. This is a diverse group of disorders. Some are neuronal lipidoses (sphingolipidoses) in which the characteristic macular sign is a cherry-red spot; this important fundus sign is described separately (see p. 47). The prototype is Tay-Sachs disease. Others are the neuronal ceroid lipofuscinoses, sometimes classified for convenience as Batten disease or Batten-Vogt syndrome. Subclassification is based on age and clinical course, and includes (1) the infantile or Haltia-Santavuori type, (2) the late infantile, Jansky-Bielschowsky form, (3) the Spielmeyer-Vogt (or Mayou) type of juvenile or later-childhood onset, and (4) Kuf disease, the adult form.

In these Batten-type cerebromacular degenerations the earliest fundus sign is often dispersion, obtunding or loss of the foveal light reflex (Fig. 18c). Definition of the macular architecture may be lost, the macula may appear dull or take on a bull's-eye appearance. In time there may be signs of generalized retinal degeneration, including pigment disorder, arteriolar attenuation and optic atrophy (Fig. 18d).

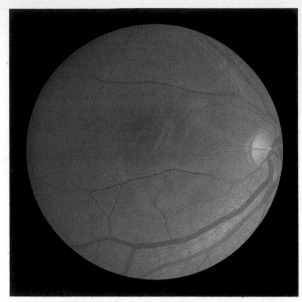

Figure 18a
Stargardt macular degeneration
Macular degeneration in this adolescent is characterized by dispersion of foveal light reflex and subtle pigment changes. Patient had no associated neurological signs.

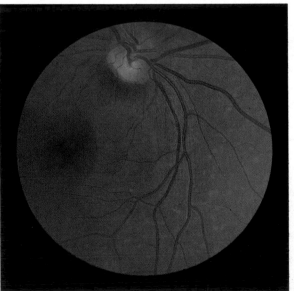

Figure 18b
Juvenile macular degeneration—flavimaculatus
This child with juvenile-onset macular degeneration also shows widespread retinal changes characteristic of fundus flavimaculatus.

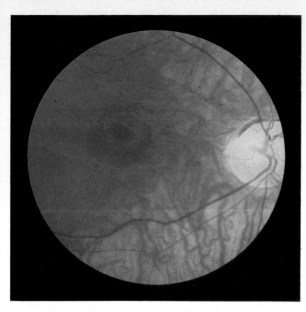

Figure 18c
Batten syndrome
In this child with progressive
cerebroretinal degeneration,
loss of foveal reflex and
bull's-eye appearance of
macula were early signs.

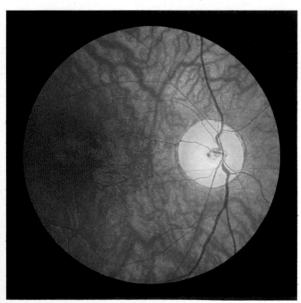

Figure 18d
*Progressive macular
degeneration*
Note marked macular
changes, arteriolar
attenuation and optic
atrophy in this child with
late-onset cerebromacular
degeneration
(lipofuscinosis).

19 PHAKOMATA

The term phakoma is derived from the Greek word for a mother spot or birthmark and is used to denote the herald lesions that occur in a number of the congenital hamartomatoses and neurocutaneous syndromes. Some of these herald lesions occur in the eye and their ophthalmoscopic appearance is often distinctive.

The characteristic ocular sign of tuberous sclerosis of Bourneville is an elevated, somewhat translucent or refractile, white to yellowish multinodular lesion of the retina or optic nervehead. The appearance of the classical lesion often is likened to that of an unripe mulberry (Fig. 19a). However, there is considerable variation in the fundus lesions of tuberous sclerosis; some are flat or only slightly elevated, dull yellow or white, and relatively smooth (Fig. 19b,c,d,e,f). The retinal lesions of tuberous sclerosis may be large or small, single or multiple, unilateral or bilateral. Histologically, they are benign astrocytic proliferations of the retina, often with cystic or calcific changes. A diligent search should be made for these tell-tale lesions in children with seizures, developmental delay and behavior disorders, with or without cutaneous signs such as adenoma sebaceum, mountain-ash leaf spots or shagreen patches.

In neurofibromatosis or von Recklinghausen disease, a retinal lesion similar to that of tuberous sclerosis may occur, but with less frequency. Another fundus sign in von Recklinghausen disease is abnormal pigmentation, likened to the café-au-lait spot of the skin. There may be disc changes, particularly optic atrophy or disc swelling of associated optic glioma, and ectopic medullation of the disc and retina occurs with somewhat increased frequency.

In addition to the fundus signs, nodular iris lesions, referred to as Lisch nodules, are important in the diagnosis of von Recklinghausen disease. There also may be neurofibromatous involvement of the lid (plexiform neuroma, ptosis) and orbit (proptosis, bony defects), or glaucoma.

In von Hippel-Lindau disease, or angiomatosis of the retina and cerebellum, the characteristic fundus lesion is a retinal hemangioblastoma. This is a globular vascular lesion that has the appearance of a toy balloon, with large paired vessels coursing to and from the lesion. In some cases the vascular changes are less conspicuous. Complications such as hemorrhage, exudation and retinal detachment may occur. The cerebellar lesion of von Hippel-Lindau disease may also produce papilledema and nystagmus, as well as ataxia.

In the Sturge-Weber syndrome of encephalofacial angiomatosis, the fundus sign is a choroidal hemangioma. This appears dark on ophthalmoscopic examination and fluoresces on angiography. Other significant fundus signs in this syndrome are tortuosity of the retinal vessels and anastamoses of the retinal veins. There may also be disc changes of intracranial hemorrhage and increased intracranial pressure. The more frequent and worrisome ocular complication of the Sturge-Weber disease, however, is glaucoma.

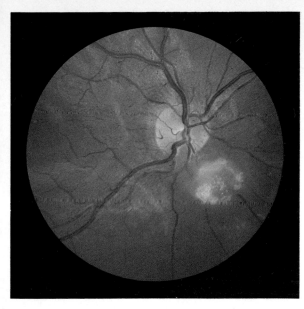

Figure 19a
Retinal phakoma
This refractile, elevated multinodular lesion is representative of classical 'mulberry' lesion of tuberous sclerosis. Patient also had typical adenoma sebaceum.

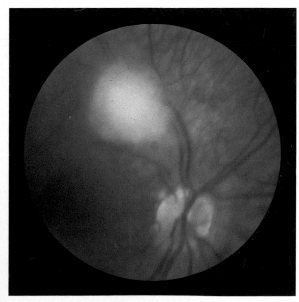

Figure 19b
Large hamartoma
Retinal phakoma in this child is quite large and smoothly elevated. Patient presented with seizures and retardation.

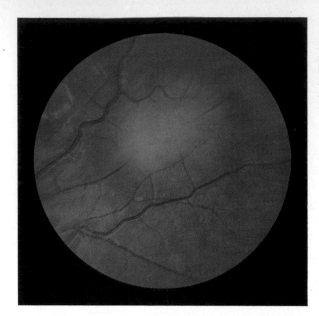

Figure 19c
Typical retinal phakoma
In many children with
tuberous sclerosis, retinal
lesions are relatively flat
and somewhat translucent,
as seen in this six-year-old
boy.

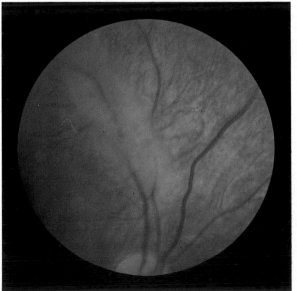

Figure 19d
Interesting variant
Translucent retinal phakoma
in this one-year-old child
with tuberous sclerosis
extends several disc
diameters along a major
retinal vessel.

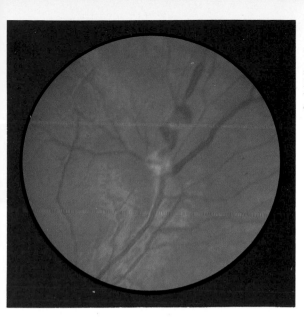

Figure 19e
*Hamartoma with vessel
abnormality*
In this child with tuberous
sclerosis a small retinal
lesion is seen in association
with sausage-like dilatation
of retinal vessels.

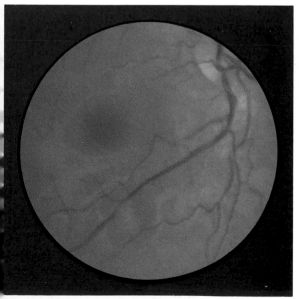

Figure 19f
*Subtle lesion of tuberous
sclerosis*
Note small yellowish
phakoma adjacent to
inferotemporal vein in this
seven-year-old child with
seizures.

Retinoblastoma is a malignant tumor that arises from the retina. It occurs in hereditary, non-hereditary, and chromosomal deletion forms. It is primarily a tumor of childhood, usually appearing before five years of age, though rarely it may occur even in adults. One or both eyes can be affected.

Retinoblastoma may be single or multiple, large or small. On ophthalmoscopic examination the smaller tumors tend to appear as translucent thickening of the retina (Fig. 20). The larger tumors usually are more opaque and white. Feeder vessels and nodular chalky foci of calcification may be evident. Seeding into the vitreous is common. Some tumors grow diffusely into the vitreous as large masses (endophytic); others extend outward (exophytic) and may produce retinal detachment.

A frequent presenting sign is leukocoria, a white or 'cat's eye' reflex in the pupil. Another common sign is strabismus—deviation of the eye secondary to impairment of vision. Some children present with signs of ocular inflammation, intra-ocular hemorrhage, glaucoma or heterochromia iridis. Differential diagnosis includes simulating conditions such as persistent hyperplastic primary vitreous, retrolental fibroplasia, retinal dysplasia, and nematode endophthalmitis.

Retinoblastoma is a vision-threatening and potentially life-threatening tumor. There may be extension into the central nervous system or metastasis to other sites, particularly bone, liver, kidney and the adrenal glands. In addition some patients with retinoblastoma are at risk for other tumors, including osteogenic sarcoma, rhabdomyosarcoma and leukemia. Some may have concurrent brain tumor, particularly pinealoma. Thus detection, or even suspicion of retinoblastoma, is reason for prompt and thorough evaluation and treatment.

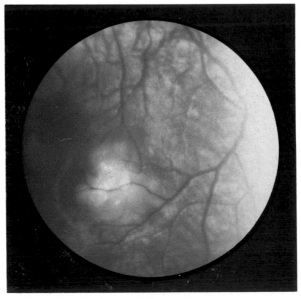

Figure 20
Retinoblastoma
Lesion, irregular in shape, is somewhat translucent, with opaque foci of calcification. Child, age nine months, also had an embryonal cell tumor of brain (suprasellar).

RETINOPATHY OF PREMATURITY
(RETROLENTAL FIBROPLASIA)

This is a complex retinal vascular disorder that occurs primarily in infants whose retinas are incompletely vascularized at birth. At highest risk are infants born prematurely, particularly those of very low birthweight and those who have been seriously ill, requiring supplemental oxygen to sustain life and to prevent brain damage. It appears that in such infants the developing or immature retinal vasculature is vulnerable to potentially adverse effects of oxygen, and possibly other factors acting singly or in combination, that may result in the pathological changes and clinically significant alterations collectively referred to as retrolental fibroplasia (RLF) or the retinopathy of prematurity (ROP).

It should be recalled that normal retinal vasculogenesis proceeds from the disc to the periphery, usually reaching the ora serrata by 38 to 44 weeks. Mesenchyme, the vascular precursor tissue, grows across the retina and gives rise to a primitive capillary meshwork; this then undergoes active modeling to form more mature capillaries, arterioles and venules.

In ROP/RLF, two major abnormal processes or phases are recognized; (1) vaso-obliteration and (2) vasoproliferation. Studies indicate that upon exposure to oxygen* or during periods of relative hyperoxia, endothelial damage, closure and obliteration of developing retinal capillaries may occur. The mesenchyme that remains and the retinal arteries and veins that have already formed may then unite through surviving capillary channels to form a shunt. On ophthalmoscopic examination one may see the abrupt termination of the retinal vasculature, with a distinct line of demarcation between the vascularized retina and the nonvascularized peripheral zone (Fig. 21a). At this site the shunt may be seen as a discrete raised gray-white structure with fan-shaped arcades of vessels emptying into it. The vessels posterior to the shunt may be dilated and tortuous. The ischemic avascular retina, peripheral to the demarcation line, generally appears pale (gray, white), translucent or opaque and thickened. Proximal to the shunt there may be small vascular tufts or neovascular membranes projecting into the vitreous. There may also be retinal hemorrhages, exudates and some degree of retinal detachment.

The acute or active changes may continue for months after birth or terminate early. Fortunately, in many cases there is spontaneous regression of the retinopathy; the change is often marked by 'pinking-up' of the shunt and the beginning of the process of vascularization of the ischemic avascular zone.

Unfortunately, in others there is progressive overgrowth of vasoproliferative tissue into the vitreous, on the surface of the retina, over the ciliary body and around the back of the lens, with progressive cicatrization. Shrinkage of tissue can result in traction on the retina, dragging or folding of the retina (Fig. 21b), or detachment of the retina, and retinal pigmentary changes. All gradations of damage may occur, with varying degrees of vision impairment. In some cases the end result is total detachment of the retina, shallowing of the anterior chamber, hemorrhage,

---

*The precise levels of oxygen and period of exposure to oxygen sufficient to produce changes in susceptible infants have yet to be determined.

inflammation, secondary angle-closure glaucoma in a blind painful eye, or phthisis. There often is leukocoria, a white pupillary reflex arising from the retrolental tissue, the organized detachment, or from a secondary cataract.

There is often associated high myopia, a little-understood complication of cicatricial RLF, and a high incidence of strabismus and amblyopia.

To be differentiated from retinopathy of prematurity is familial exudative vitreoretinopathy, a disorder of the vitreous and retina that occurs as an autosomal dominant condition. It is characterized by the presence of organized membranes (often containing large blood vessels) in the vitreous, peripheral retinal exudation (subretinal and intraretinal), and in some cases localized retinal detachment and recurrent vitreous hemorrhages. The ocular changes are progressive and tend to run a downhill course.

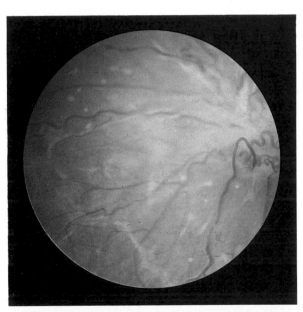

Figure 21a
Active ROP
Retinal edema and tortuosity of retinal vessels are evident.

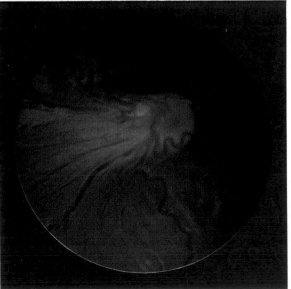

Figure 21b
'Dragged disc'
This picture is typical of cicatricial RLF. There is dragging of retina and retinal vessels to temporal side of disc.

HYPERTENSIVE RETINOPATHY

The hallmark of hypertensive retinopathy is vasoconstriction. The vascular tone of the retinal artery increases by a process of autoregulation in response to the rise in blood pressure. On ophthalmoscopic examination one may see generalized arteriolar narrowing, focal arteriolar constriction ('spasm') with irregularity in the caliber of the vessels, and arterial tortuosity (Fig. 22a). Associated vessel damage and disruption of the blood-retinal barrier may occur, leading to leakage of plasma and formed blood elements in the retina. Clinically one may see retinal edema, hemorrhages and exudates (Fig. 22b). The hemorrhages typically are flame-shaped or splinter hemorrhages, as the extravasation of blood occurs primarily in the nerve-fiber layer. The exudates or edema residues appear yellow; those in the macula may form a star-shaped figure. In addition there may be superficial white spots called 'cotton-wool spots'; these are the result of focal ischemia and swelling of retinal-nerve fibers.

In time arteriolar sclerosis may occur. This is manifested by changes in the color of the arterioles, and changes in the arteriovenous crossings. As the vessel wall becomes 'harder' or 'thicker', the ophthalmoscopic reflection from the wall increases and the visibility of the blood column decreases; as sclerosis progresses the arteriole may take on a copper-wire appearance, or ultimately a silver-wire appearance. At arteriovenous crossings one may see obscuration of the venous blood column, deflection or change in the course of the vessels as they cross and, in some cases, signs of venous impedance (dilatation, tortuosity) distal to the crossing.

Another important manifestation of hypertension is hypertensive disc edema, characterized by swelling of the nervehead and blurring of the disc margins. This may occur with or without increased intracranial pressure of hypertensive encephalopathy. The pathogenesis is unclear, but alteration in the circulation to the optic nervehead and changes in tissue pressure and axoplasmic flow may occur in hypertension. Ischemia has been implicated as a factor.

In addition to the retinovascular and disc signs of hypertension there may be clinical signs of hypertensive choroidopathy, particularly in acute hypertension and in relatively young individuals. One may see changes in the retinal-pigment layer as a result of occlusive changes in the underlying choriocapillaries. Clinically, these appear as yellowish spots, or pigmented spots with depigmented halos, referred to as Elschnig spots.

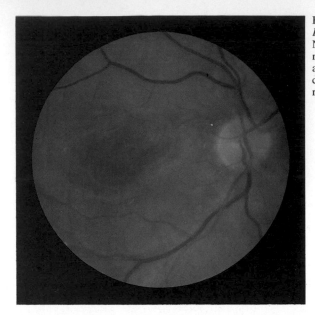

Figure 22a
Hypertensive retinopathy
Note generalized and focal
narrowing of retinal
arterioles, arteriovenous
crossing abnormality and
retinal edema.

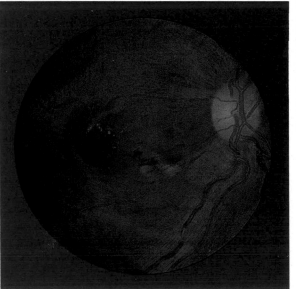

Figure 22b
Hypertensive retinopathy
In this child there are
marked hypertensive
changes including multiple
retinal hemorrhages,
exudates and prominent
alterations of the arterioles
and veins. (The fundus is
that of a black child; hence
the dark slate hue.)

DIABETIC RETINOPATHY

The retinal manifestations of diabetes mellitus are classified as (1) simple or non-proliferative retinopathy, and (2) proliferative, the more severe type.

Non-proliferative or background retinopathy is characterized by venous dilatation, micro-aneurysms, retinal hemorrhages, exudates, cytoid bodies, and retinal edema (Fig. 23). The micro-aneurysms appear as tiny red dots; they often are the first detectable finding. The retinal hemorrhages may be of both the deep (intraretinal) dot and blot type, and the more superficial (nerve-fiber layer) splinter or flame-shaped type. The exudates tend to be deep and appear waxy. Cytoid bodies, descriptively referred to as cotton-wool spots, are superficial nerve-fiber infarcts. These background changes may wax and wane.

Proliferative retinopathy is characterized by neovascularization and proliferation of connective tissue on the retina and into the vitreous, often with vision-threatening complications such as retinal and vitreous hemorrhages, cicatrization, traction and retinal detachment. Rubeosis (abnormal vascularization of the iris) and secondary glaucoma may develop.

The incidence of diabetic retinopathy increases with duration of disease and with age. The incidence is low within the first five years of disease and increases thereafter. It is rare in prepubescent children, but its prevalence increases after puberty, rising noticeably after age 15 years. Examination of the fundus is important in the care of youngsters with diabetes.

In addition to retinal changes, patients with juvenile-onset diabetes may develop optic neuropathy, characterized by optic-disc edema with blurring of vision. They also may develop cataracts, sometimes of rapid onset.

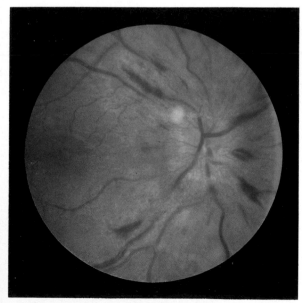

Figure 23
Diabetic retinopathy
Note multiple dot-like mirco-aneurysms, irregular dilatation of veins, splinter and flame-shaped hemorrhages, peripapillary cotton-wool spot and retinal edema. This girl's retinopathy developed at 16 years of age.

In various types of hyperlipoproteinemia there may be visible alteration in the color of the plasma. In some cases this change can be detected ophthalmoscopically, the blood column of the retinal vessels having a pale or creamy appearance (Fig. 24a); the term lipemia retinalis is used to describe this fundus sign.

The clinical picture can be dramatic, the creaminess being evident in vessels throughout the fundus; the fundus background may even appear pale, pink, or salmon colored. In some cases the change can be detected only in the smaller and more peripheral vessels where the blood column is thinner. Visibility of the lipemia may also vary with the transparency of the vessel walls, and the clarity of the ocular media.

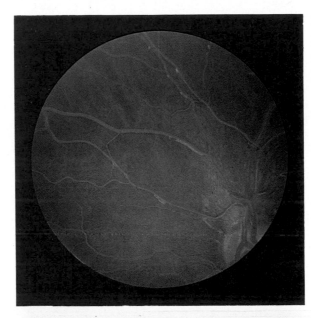

Figure 24a
Lipemia retinalis
Creamy alteration of blood column of retinal vessels is evident in this young girl with hyperlipidemia.

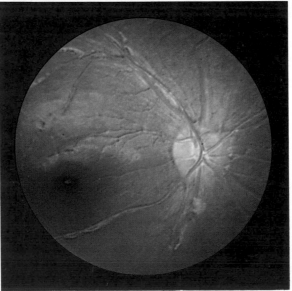

Figure 24b
Lipemia retinalis
Note milky pallor of fundus in addition to whitish lamination of blood-vessel column. This nine-year-old girl had hyperlipidemia and diabetes mellitus.

Lipemia retinalis is related to the level of triglycerides. It may occur in types I, III, IV or V hyperlipoproteinemia. In children with lipemia retinalis, type I (lipoprotein lipase deficiency) is the primary consideration; symptoms usually appear in the first decade. Lipemia retinalis may also be associated with diabetes mellitus (Fig. 24b).

Other ocular signs occurring with the various forms of hyperlipoproteinemia include xanthomas and corneal arcus.

Historically, this appellation has been used to denote the white-centered retinal hemorrhages seen in patients with subacute bacterial endocarditis, which were believed to be caused by septic emboli.

Similar in appearance, however, are the white-centered hemorrhages that occur in leukemia and a number of other systemic and ocular conditions, including ischemia, anoxia and anemia, diabetic and hypertensive retinopathy, and trauma, notably birth trauma and child abuse, to name just a few (Fig. 25). The white center in these hemorrhages is a fibrin thrombus.

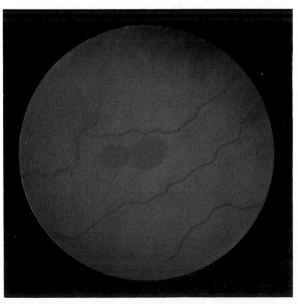

Figure 25
White-centered hemorrhage
Retinal hemorrhage with white center seen in this infant was due to trauma (child abuse).

The fundus signs of leukemia include dilatation, engorgement and tortuosity of the retinal veins, sheathing of the retinal vessels, retinal hemorrhages, exudates, cotton-wool spots, and nodular retinal infiltrates (Fig. 26). There may also be optic-nerve changes.

The dilatation of the veins is often irregular, producing a sausage-like appearance. The blood column may appear not only broad but pale, reflecting the increased white blood-cell content and the decreased red blood-cell content. In some cases there may be signs of venous obstruction.

Retinal hemorrhages are a frequent sign. They occur in all types of leukemia and are often present at the time of presentation or diagnosis. The retinal hemorrhages of leukemia are usually located in the posterior pole and in relationship to the retinal vessels. They may be of the superficial flame-shaped type, often with a white center, or of the deeper intraretinal round or blot type. Sometimes they are of the subhyaloid or so-called preretinal type, forming a fluid level and having the configuration of a boat keel. In some cases there is extravasation of blood into the vitreous, affecting vision and impairing visualization of the fundus.

Perivascular sheathing appears as a gray or white line along the vessel wall, resulting from diapedesis of the cells. There may also be localized aggregates of white cells, commonly referred to as leukemic nodules. These are to be differentiated from the exudates and cotton-wool patches (nerve-fiber infarcts) that may occur in leukemia.

With leukemic infiltration of the optic nerve one may see swelling of the nervehead, or a proliferative lesion, appearing as a fluffy or grayish mass protruding from the disc. With intracranial involvement, there may be papilledema of increased intracranial pressure.

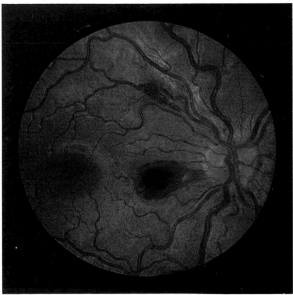

Figure 26
Leukemic retinopathy
In this child with acute lymphocytic leukemia, venous dilatation and tortuosity, and retinal hemorrhages are principal signs. Note small white spot in retinal hemorrhage, temporal to the disc.

The fundus signs, though frequent, are but a portion of the whole spectrum of leukemic ophthalmopathy. Other important manifestations are uveal involvement, notably iris infiltrates, hyphemia (bleeding into the anterior chamber), hypopyon (creamy layering of cells in the aqueous), lid, lacrymal and conjunctival infiltrates, and orbital masses. In addition one may see ocular complications of radiation therapy or evidence of ocular infection by opportunistic organisms.

RETINAL TELANGIECTASIS

Retinal telangiectasis, also referred to as Leber's miliary aneurysms, is a developmental vascular anomaly characterized by ophthalmoscopically visible, focal saccular dilatations of intraretinal capillaries, arterioles or venules (Fig. 27). The lesions usually are monocular, infrequently bilateral. There is propensity for temporal retinal location, though any area of the retina may be involved. The lesions occur in childhood and tend to be found primarily in adolescent males. The condition occasionally is familial. As a rule there are no regularly associated systemic lesions, though isolated instances of other abnormalities have been reported.

The extent and natural course of retinal telangiectasis is variable, but there is a tendency to intraretinal and subretinal exudation. This may lead to massive exudative detachment of the retina, often having a yellowish color, with attendant disturbance of vision, a condition referred to as Coats' disease. Such lesions may require treatment; ophthalmological evaluation and careful follow-up are indicated.

Not to be confused with congenital retinal telangiectasis is cavernous hemangioma of the retina, a hamartomatous condition characterized by a sessile hemangiomatous mass composed of clusters of saccular aneurysms of retinal vessels having the appearance of grapes projecting from the surface of the retina. It has been suggested that cavernous hemangioma of the retina and brain may occur together, and there may also be associated cutaneous lesions.

Also to be distinguished from retinal telangiectasis are aneurysmal changes of retina vessels that may occur with diabetes, venous stasis, macroglobulinemia, sickle-cell disease, or in association with angiomatosis retinae (von Hippel-Lindau disease, see p. 52), or racemose angioma, a very rare condition which may occur in association with arteriovenous malformation of the brain (Wyburn-Mason syndrome).

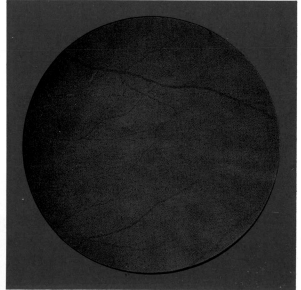

Figure 27
Retinal telangiectasis
Note multiple small grape-like aneurysmal lesions in the temporal fundus. Patient was an adolescent male referred for evaluation of learning disability. There were no associated systemic or neurological abnormalities.

Tortuosity of the retinal arterioles may occur as a benign congenital variant (Fig. 28). It may also occur as a familial disorder, and in some cases it may be associated with recurrent retinal hemorrhages and visual symptoms. The hemorrhages may be spontaneous or related to physical exertion. Usually there are no associated systemic abnormalities, though there may be a history of hemorrhages in other parts of the body.

To be differentiated from congenital retinal tortuosity is the tortuosity that may occur with hypertension, and this is an important sign in children with coarctation of the aorta. Also to be considered in the differential diagnosis of tortuosity are leukemia, polycythemia, macroglobulinemia, cryglobulinemia, sickle-cell disease, mucopolysaccharidosis (specifically Maroteaux-Lamy syndrome), and Fabry disease. Not to be confused with benign congenital retinal tortuosity are the retinal signs of Wyburn-Mason syndrome (racemose angioma of the retina and arteriovenous malformations of the brain) and of von Hippel-Lindau disease (angiomatosis retinae et cerebellae).

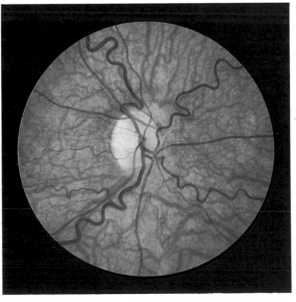

Figure 28
Retinal arteriolar tortuosity
Tortuosity of retinal artery in this child is a normal developmental variant.

PREPAPILLARY VASCULAR LOOPS

In some individuals vascular loops may be seen projecting from the disc into the vitreous. The configuration may vary from that of a simple hairpin turn to a spiral, corkscrew, or figure-eight twist (Fig. 29). Some are surrounded by a sheath of whitish glial tissue. Some may be seen to pulsate. These are congenital anomalies. They are more often arterial than venous. They may be unilateral or bilateral.

In most cases prepapillary vascular loops present no problem, occurring just as interesting incidental findings in otherwise normal eyes. Occasionally, however, they may be associated with retinal vascular obstruction or hemorrhage.

Not to be confused with these simple congenital prepapillary vascular loops are more complex vascular anomalies, such as racemose angiomas that may be associated with arteriovenous malformations of the brain.

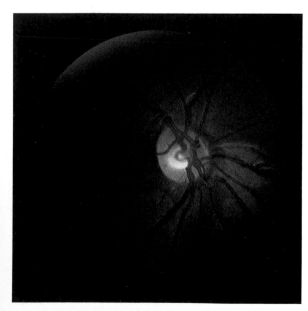

Figure 29
Prepapillary vascular loop
Note twisted loop of vessel projecting from disc. This is a developmental variant with no associated vascular or neurological signs in this child.

Hypopigmentation of the fundus is a not-uncommon finding and presents a number of diagnostic possibilities. Though marked hypopigmentation of the fundus may be seen as a normal developmental variant in many blond individuals, especially in infants and young children, pigment deficiency can be an important manifestation of metabolic disease. Of primary importance in the differential diagnosis of pathological fundus hypopigmentation are the various forms of albinism.

In oculocutaneous albinism there is generalized hypopigmentation of the skin, hair and eyes. The iris typically is pale blue or gray and translucent. The fundus appears pale and red-streaked owing to absence of background pigmentation and increased visibility of the underlying sclera and choroidal vasculature (Fig. 30a). In addition there is hypoplasia of the macula—it appears flat with poor definition of the ganglion-cell ring and foveal light-reflex, and the disc also may appear pale, grayish and somewhat hypoplastic. Vision is subnormal, there is nystagmus, and the patient is sensitive to light. High refractive errors and strabismus are frequent associated findings.

Tyrosinase negative and tyrosinase positive forms of oculocutaneous albinism can be differentiated; these are recessive. An Amish or yellow variant, having a different enzyme defect, also occurs; ocular signs are similar and persist throughout life, though some skin color develops.

Incomplete forms of albinism also occur and an important example is ocular albinism. In this condition hypopigmentation is limited to the eye. The condition is most commonly x-linked and pigment disorder of the fundus may be seen in carrier females.

Important syndromes associated with various forms of albinism are the Hermansky-Pudlak syndrome, the Chediak-Higashi syndrome, and the Cross syndrome. The Hermansky-Pudlak syndrome is an autosomal recessive condition characterized by oculocutaneous albinism and a hemorrhagic diathesis. The Chediak-Higashi syndrome is characterized by incomplete oculocutaneous albinisim, neutropenia, and susceptibility to pyogenic infections. The Cross syndrome is characterized by hypopigmentation, gingival fibromatosis, spasticity, athetoid movements, and microphthalmos.

To be considered in the differential diagnosis of partial albinism is Waardenburg syndrome; this autosomal dominant condition is characterized primarily by poliosis, heterochromia, telecanthus, and hearing impairment.

It is of interest that children with cystinosis or Menke's trichopoliodystrophy may also have a markedly hypopigmented or albinotic fundus (Fig. 30b).

To be differentiated from the developmental disorders affecting pigmentation are the degenerative diseases characterized by loss of pigment, such as retinitis pigmentosa and choroideremia.

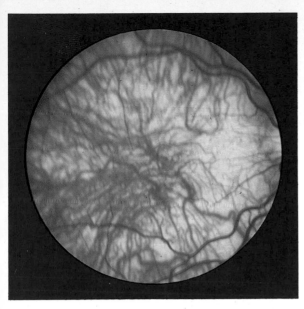

Figure 30a
Albinism
This child with oculocutaneous albinism shows the classical findings of generalized hypopigmentation of the fundus with increased visibility of the choroidal vascular pattern.

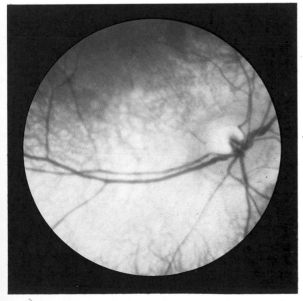

Figure 30b
Albinotic fundus
Marked hypopigmentation of fundus seen here is in a child with Menke's trichopoliodystrophy, a complex metabolic neurodegencrative disease.

This disorder is characterized by the presence of multiple yellow-white spots in the retina in association with congenital stationary night-blindness. The fundus spots are small (about the size of a second-order arteriole) and extend from the posterior pole to the periphery (Fig. 31a,b).

To be distinguished from fundus albipunctatus is retinitis punctata albescens, a degenerative disorder characterized by progressive visual-field loss, retinal pigmentary changes and arteriolar attenuation.

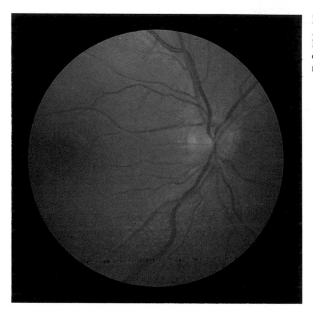

Figure 31a
Fundus albipunctatus
Note punctate yellow spots of retina. Retinal vessels are normal.

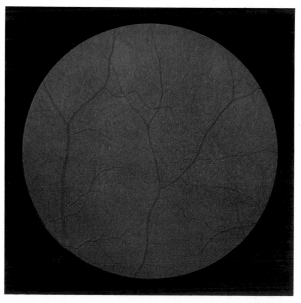

Figure 31b
Fundus albipunctatus
Typical yellow punctate lesions are seen throughout periphery.

SELECTED READING

Papilledema
Barr C. C., Glaser, J. S., Blankenship, G. (1980) 'Acute disc swelling in juvenile diabetes. Clinical profile and natural history of 12 cases.' *Archives of Ophthalmology,* **98,** 2185-2192.
Billson F. A., Hudson, R. L. (1975) 'Surgical treatment of chronic papillodema in children.' *British Journal of Ophthalmology,* **59,** 92-95.
Buchheit, W. A., Burton, C., Haag, B., Shaw, D. (1969) 'Papilledema and idiopathic intracranial hypertension. Report of a familial occurrence.' *New England Journal of Medicine,* **280,** 938-942.
Hayreh, S. S. (1977) 'Optic disc edema in raised intracranial pressure. V. Pathogenesis.' *Archives of Ophthalmology,* **95,** 1553-1565.
Hayreh, S. S. (1977) 'Optic disc edema in raised intracranial pressure. VI. Associated visual disturbances and their pathogenesis.' *Archives of Ophthalmology,* **95,** 1566-1579.
Pavan, P. R., Aiello, L. M., Wafai, M. Z., Briones, J. C., Sebestyen, J. G., Bradbury, M. J. (1980) 'Optic disc edema in juvenile-onset diabetes.' *Archives of Ophthalmology,* **96,** 2193-2195.
Rosenberg, M. A., Savino, P. J., Glaser, J. S. (1979) 'A clinical analysis of pseudopapilledema. I. Population, laterality, acuity, refractive error, ophthalmoscopic characteristics, and coincident disease.' *Archives of Ophthalmology,* **97,** 65-70.
Savino, P. J., Glaser, J. S., Rosenberg, M. A. (1979) 'A clinical analysis of pseudopapilledema. II. Visual field defects.' *Archives of Ophthalmology,* **97,** 71-75.

Optic neuritis
Frey, T. (1973) 'Optic neuritis in children. Infectious mononucleosis as an etiology.' *Documenta Ophthalmologica,* **34,** 183-188.
Godel, V., Nemet, P., Lazar, M. (1980) 'Chloramphenicol optic neuropathy.' *Archives of Ophthalmology,* **98,** 1417-1421.
Harley, R. D., Huang, N. N., Macri, C. H., Green, W. R. (1970) 'Optic neuritis and optic atrophy following chloramphenicol in cystic fibrosis patients.' *Transactions of the American Academy of Ophthalmology and Otolaryngology,* **74,** 1011-1031.
Kazarian, E. L., Gager, W. E. (1978) 'Optic neuritis complicating measles, mumps, and rubella vaccination.' *American Journal of Ophthalmology,* **86,** 544-547.
Kennedy, C., Carroll, F. D. (1960) 'Optic neuritis in children.' *Archives of Ophthalmology,* **63,** 747-755.
Kennedy, C., Carter, S. (1961) 'Relation of optic neuritis to multiple sclerosis in children.' *Pediatrics,* **28,** 377-387.
Meadows, S. R. (1969) 'Retrobulbar and optic neuritis in childhood and adolescence.' *Transactions of the Ophthalmological Society of the United Kingdom,* **89,** 603-638.
Selbst, R. G., Selhorst, J. B., Harrison, J. W., Myer, E. C. (1983) 'Parainfectious optic neuritis. Report and review following varicella.' *Archives of Neurology,* **40,** 347-350.
Smith, J. L., Hoyt, W. F., Susac, J. D. (1973) 'Ocular fundus in acute Leber optic neuropathy.' *Archives of Ophthalmology,* **90,** 349-354.
Strong, L. E., Henderson, J. W., Gangitano, J. L. (1974) 'Bilateral retrobulbar neuritis secondary to mumps.' *American Journal of Ophthalmology,* **78,** 331-332.

Optic atrophy
Blodi, F. C. (1957) 'Developmental anomalies of the skull affecting the eye.' *Archives of Ophthalmology,* **57,** 593-610.
Davis, W. H., Nevins, R. C., Elliott, J. H. (1972) 'Optic atrophy after ocular contusion.' *American Journal of Ophthalmology,* **73,** 278-280.
Fishman, M. L., Bean, S. C., Cogan, D. G. (1976) 'Optic atrophy following prophylactic chemotherapy and cranial radiation for acute lymphocytic leukemia.' *American Journal of Ophthalmology,* **82,** 571-576.
Hoyt, C. S. (1980) 'Autosomal dominant optic atrophy. A spectrum of disability.' *Ophthalmology,* **87,** 245-251.
Kline, L. B., Glaser, J. S. (1979) 'Dominant optic atrophy. The clinical profile.' *Archives of Ophthalmology,* **97,** 1680-1686.
Kollarits, C. R., Pinheiro, M. L., Swann, E. R., Marcus, D. F., Corrie, W. S. (1979) 'The autosomal dominant syndrome of progressive optic atrophy and congenital deafness.' *American Journal of Ophthalmology,* **87,** 789-792.
Nikoskelainen, E., Sogg, R. I., Rosenthal, A. R., Friberg, T. R., Dorfman, L. J. (1977) 'The early phase in Leber hereditary optic atrophy.' *Archives of Ophthalmology,* **95,** 969-978.
Schwartz, J. F., Chutorian, A. M., Evans, R. A., Carter, S. (1964) 'Optic atrophy in childhood.' *Pediatrics,* **34,** 670-679.
Wybar, K. C. (1972) 'Acquired optic atrophy in early childhood.' *In* Cant, J. S. (Ed.) *The Optic Nerve.* London: Henry Kimpton; St. Louis: C. V. Mosby. pp. 12-18.

Optic-cup enlargement

Armaly, M. F. (1967) 'Genetic determination of cup/disc ratio of the optic nerve.' *Archives of Ophthalmology*, **78**, 35-43.

Armaly, M. F. (1969) 'The optic cup in the normal eye. I. Cup width, depth, vessel displacement, ocular tension and outflow facility.' *American Journal of Ophthalmology*, **68**, 401-407.

Khodadoust, A. A. Ziai, M., Biggs, S. L. (1968) 'Optic disc in normal newborns.' *American Journal of Ophthalmology*, **66**, 502-504.

Richardson, K. T., Shaffer, R. N. (1966) 'Optic-nerve cupping in congenital glaucoma.' *American Journal of Ophthalmology*, **62**, 507-509.

Robin, A. L., Quigley, H. A., Pollack, I. P., Maumenee, A. E., Maumenee, I. H. (1979) 'An analysis of visual acuity, visual fields, and disk cupping in childhood glaucoma.' *American Journal of Ophthalmology*, **88**, 847-858.

Optic-nerve pits

Brown, G. C., Shields, J. A., Goldberg, R. E. (1980) 'Congenital pits of the optic nerve head. II. Clinical studies in humans.' *Ophthalmology*, **87**, 51-65.

Pfaffenbach, D. D., Walsh, F. B. (1972) 'Central pit of the optic disk.' *American Journal of Ophthalmology*, **73**, 102-106.

Optic-nerve hypoplasia

Brook, C. G. D., Sanders, M. D., Hoare, R. D. (1972) 'Septo-optic dysplasia.' *British Medical Journal*, **3**, 811-813.

Krause-Brucker, W., Gardner, D. W. (1980) 'Optic nerve hypoplasia associated with absent septum pellucidum and hypopituitarism.' *American Journal of Ophthalmology*, **89**, 113-120.

Layman, P. R., Anderson, D. R., Flynn, J. T. (1974) 'Frequent occurrence of hypoplastic optic disks in patients with aniridia.' *American Journal of Ophthalmology*, **77**, 513-516.

Mosier, M. A., Lieberman, M. F., Green, W. R., Knox, D. L. (1978) 'Hypoplasia of the optic nerve.' *Archives of Ophthalmology*, **96**, 1437-1442.

Petersen, R. A., Walton, D. S. (1977) 'Optic nerve hypoplasia with good visual acuity and visual field defects. A study of children of diabetic mothers.' *Archives of Ophthalmology*, **95**, 254-258.

Skarf, B., Hoyt, C. S. (1984) 'Optic nerve hypoplasia in children. Association with anomalies of the endocrine and CNS.' *Archives of Ophthalmology*, **102**, 62-67.

Walton, D. S., Robb, R. M. (1970) 'Optic nerve hypoplasia. A report of 20 cases.' *Archives of Ophthalmology*, **84**, 572-578

Weiter, J. J., McLean, I. W., Zimmerman, L. E. (1977) 'Aplasia of the optic nerve and disk.' *American Journal of Ophthalmology*, **83**, 569-576.

Tilted disc

Graham, M. V., Wakefield, G. J. (1973) 'Bitemporal visual field defects associated with anomalies of the optic discs.' *British Journal of Ophthalmology*, **57**, 307-314.

Hittner, H. M., Borda, R. P., Justice, J. (1981) 'X-linked recessive congenital stationary night blindness, myopia, and tilted discs.' *Journal of Pediatric Ophthalmoplegia and Strabismus*, **18**, 15-20.

Young, S. E., Walsh, F. B., Knox, D. L. (1976) 'The tilted disk syndrome.' *American Journal of Ophthalmology*, **82**, 16-23.

Optic-disc drusen

Frisén, L., Schöldström, G., Svendsen, P. (1978) 'Drusen in the optic nerve head. Verification by computerized tomography.' *Archives of Ophthalmology*, **96**, 1611-1614.

Harris, M. J., Fine, S. L., Owens, S. L. (1981) 'Hemorrhagic complications of optic nerve drusen.' *American Journal of Ophthalmology*, **92**, 70-76.

Sanders, T. E., Gay, A. J., Newman, M. (1971) 'Hemorrhagic complications of drusen of the optic disk.' *American Journal of Ophthalmology*, **71**, (Suppl.) 204-217.

Spencer, W. H. (1978) 'Drusen of the optic disk and aberrant axoplasmic transport.' *American Journal of Ophthalmology*, **85**, 1-12.

Tso, M. O. M. (1981) 'Pathology and pathogenesis of drusen of the optic nervehead.' *Ophthalmology*, **88**, 1066-1080.

Persistent Bergmeister papilla

Lloyd, R. I. (1940) 'Variations in the development and regression of Bergmeister's papilla and the hyaloid artery.' *Transactions of the American Ophthalmological Society*, **38**, 326-332.

Roth, A. M., Foos, R. Y. (1972) 'Surface structure of the optic nerve head. Epipapillary membranes.' *American Journal of Ophthalmology*, **74**, 977-985.

74

Persistent hyperplastic primary vitreous (PHPV)
Brown, G. C., Gonder, J., Levin, A. (1984) 'Persistence of the primary vitreous in association with the morning glory disc anomaly.' *Journal of Pediatric Ophthalmology and Strabismus*, **21**, 5-7.
Federman, J., Shields, J. A., Altman, B., Koller, H. (1982) 'The surgical and non-surgical management of persistent hyperplastic primary vitreous.' *Ophthalmology*, **89**, 20-24.
Goldberg, M. F., Mafee, M. (1983) 'Computed tomography for diagnosis of persistent hyperplastic primary vitreous (PHPV).' *Ophthalmology*, **90**, 442-451.
Haddad, R , Font, R. L,, Reeser, F. (1978) 'Persistent hyperplastic primary vitreous: a clinico-pathologic study of 62 cases and review of the literature.' *Survey of Ophthalmology*, **23**, 123-124.
Pruett, R. C., Schepens, C. L. (1970) 'Posterior hyperplastic primary vitreous.' *American Journal of Ophthalmology*, **69**, 535-543.
Reese, A. B. (1955) 'Persistent hyperplastic primary vitreous.' *American Journal of Ophthalmology*, **40**, 317-331.

Myelinated nerve fibers
Holland, P. M., Anderson, B. (1976) 'Myelinated nerve fibers and severe myopia.' *American Journal of Ophthalmology*, **81**, 597-599.
Straatsma, B. R., Heckenlively, J. R., Foos, R. Y., Shahinian, J. K. (1979) 'Myelinated retinal nerve fibers associated with ipsilateral myopia, ambylopia and strabismus.' *American Journal of Ophthalmology*, **88**, 506-510.
Straatsma, B. R., Foos, R. Y., Heckenlively, J. R., Taylor, G. N. (1981) 'Myelinated retinal nerve fibers.' *American Journal of Ophthalmology*, **91**, 25-38.

Peripapillary crescents
Shields, M. B. (1980) 'Gray crescent in the optic nerve head.' *American Journal of Ophthalmology*, **89**, 238-244.

Colobomata
Francois J. (1968) 'Colobomatous malformations of the ocular globe.' *International Ophthalmological Clinics*, **8**, 797-817.
Goldhammer, Y., Smith, J. L. (1975) 'Optic nerve anomalies in basal encephalocele.' *Archives of Ophthalmology*, **93**, 115-118.
Hittner, H. M., Desmond, M. M., Montgomery, J. R. (1976) 'Optic nerve manifestations of human congenital cytomegalovirus infection.' *American Journal of Ophthalmology*, **81**, 661-665.
James, P. M. L., Karseras, A. G., Wybar, K. C. (1974) 'Systemic associations of uveal coloboma.' *British Journal of Ophthalmology*, 58, 917-921.
Kindler, P. (1970) 'Morning glory syndrome. Unusual congenital optic disc anomaly.' *American Journal of Ophthalmology*, **69**, 376-384.
Koenig, S. B., Naidich, T. P., Lissner, G. (1982) 'The morning glory syndrome associated with sphenoidal encephalocoele.' *Ophthalmology*, **89**, 1368-1373.
Pagon, R. A., Graham, J. M., Zonana, J., Young, S. L. (1981) 'Coloboma congenital heart disease, and choanal atresia with multiple anomalies. CHARGE association.' *Journal of Pediatrics*, **99**, 223-227.
Savell, J., Cook, J. R. (1976) 'Optic nerve coloboma of autosomal-dominant heredity.' *Archives of Ophthalmology*, **94**, 395-400.

Chorioretinitis
Asbell, P. A., Vermund, S. H., Hopelot, A. J. (1982) 'Presumed toxoplasmic retinochoroiditis in four siblings.' *American Journal of Ophthalmology*, **94**, 656-663.
Charles, N. C., Bennett, T. W., Margolis, J. I. (1977) 'Ocular pathology of the congenital varicella syndrome.' *Archives of Ophthalmology*, **95**, 2034-2037.
Chumbley, L. C., Kearns, T. P. (1972) 'Retinopathy of sarcoidosis.' *American Journal of Ophthalmology*, **73**, 123-131.
Cibis, G. W., Flynn, J. T., Davis, E. B. (1978) 'Herpes simplex retinitis.' *Archives of Ophthalmology*, **96**, 299-302.
Cogan, D. G. (1977) 'Immunosuppression and eye disease.' *American Journal of Ophthalmology*, **83**, 777-788.
Cogan, D. G., Kuwabara, T., Young, G. F., Knox, D. L. (1964) 'Herpes simplex retinopathy in an infant.' *Archives of Ophthalmology*, **72**, 641-645.
Cox, F., Meyer, D., Hughes, W. T. (1975) 'Cytomegalovirus in tears from patients with normal eyes and with acute cytomegalovirus chorioretinitis.' *American Journal of Ophthalmology*, **80**, 817-824.
Desmonts, G., Couvreue, J. (1974) 'Toxoplasmosis in pregnancy and its transmission to the fetus.' *Bulletin of the New York Academy of Medicine*, **50**, 146-159.

Duguid, I. M. (1961) 'Features of ocular infestation by *Toxocara*.' *British Journal of Ophthalmology*, **45**, 789-796.

Fine, S. L., Owens, S. L., Haller, J. A., Knox, D. L., Patz, A. (1981) 'Choroidal neovascularization as a late complication of ocular toxoplasmosis.' *American Journal of Ophthalmology*, **91**, 318-322.

Gould, H., Kaufman, H. E. (1961) 'Sarcoid of the fundus.' *Archives of Ophthalmology*, **65**, 453-456.

Hagler, W. S., Walters, P. V., Naumias, A. J. (1969) 'Ocular involvement in neonatal Herpes simplex virus infection.' *Archives of Ophthalmology*, **82**, 169-176.

Hogan, M. J., Kimura, S. J., Spencer, W. H. (1965) 'Visceral larva migrans and peripheral retinitis.' *Journal of the American Medical Association*, **194**, 1345-1347.

Knox, D. L., (1983) 'Disorders of the uveal tract.' *In* Harley, R. D. (Ed.) *Pediatric Ophthalmology, 2nd Edn.* Philadelphia: W. B. Saunders.

Lonn, L. I. (1972) 'Neonatal cytomegalic inclusion disease chorioretinitis.' *Archives of Ophthalmology*, **88**, 434-438.

Martyn, L. J., Lischner, H. W., Pileggi, A. J., Harley, R. D. (1972) 'Chorioretinal lesions in familial chronic granulomatous disease of childhood.' *American Journal of Ophthalmology*, **72**, 403-418.

Molk, R. (1983) 'Ocular toxocaiasis: a review of the literature.' *Annals of Ophthalmology*, **15**, 216-231.

Pollard, Z. F. (1979) 'Ocular toxocara in siblings of two families. Diagnosis confirmed by Elisa test.' *Archives of Ophthalmology*, **97**, 2319-2320.

Smith, M. E., Zimmerman, L. E., Harley, R. D. (1966) 'Ocular involvement in congenital cytomegalic inclusion disease.' *Archives of Ophthalmology*, **76**, 696-699.

Smith, R. E., Ganley, J. P. (1972) 'Presumed ocular histoplasmosis. I. Histoplasmin skin test sensitivity in cases identified during a community survey.' *Archives of Ophthalmology*, **87**, 245-250.

Zimmerman, L. (1961) 'Ocular pathology of toxoplasmosis.' *Survey of Ophthalmology*, **6**, 832-839.

'Salt and pepper' retinopathy

Bateman, J. B., Riedner, E. D., Levin, L. S., Maumenee, I. N. (1980) 'Heterogeneity of retinal degeneration and hearing impairment syndromes.' *American Journal of Ophthalmology*, **90**, 755-767.

Boniuk, M., Zimmerman, L. E. (1967) 'Ocular pathology in the rubella syndrome.' *Archives of Ophthalmology*, **77**, 455-473.

Deutman, A. F., Grizzard, W. S. (1978) 'Rubella retinopathy and subretinal neovascularization.' *American Journal of Ophthalmology*, **85**, 82-87.

Hertzberg, R. (1968) 'Twenty-five-year follow-up of ocular defects in congenital rubella.' *American Journal of Ophthalmology*, **66**, 269-271.

Krill, A. E. (1967) 'The retinal disease of rubella.' *American Journal of Ophthalmology*, **77**, 445-449.

Scheie, H. G., Morse, P. H. (1972) 'Rubeola retinopathy.' *Archives of Ophthalmology*, **88**, 341-344.

Wong, V. G. (1976) 'Ocular manifestations in cystinosis.' *Birth Defects. Original Article Series*, **XII**, 181-186.

Pigmentary retinal degeneration

Bateman, J. B., Riedner, E. D., Levin, L. S., Maumenee, I. H. (1980) 'Heterogeneity of retinal degeneration and hearing impairment syndromes.' *American Journal of Ophthalmology*, **90**, 755-767.

Berson, E. L., Rosner, B., Simonoff, E. (1980) 'Risk factors for genetic typing and detection in retinitis pigmentosa.' *American Journal of Ophthalmology*, **89**, 763-775.

Edwards, W. C., Grizzard, W. S. (1981) 'Tapeto-retinal degeneration associated with renal disease.' *Journal of Pediatric Ophthalmology and Strabismus*, **18**, 55-57.

Eller, W. E., Brown, G. C. (1984) 'Retinal disorders of childhood.' *American Journal of Ophthalmology*, **98**, 1099-1101.

Fishman, G. A., Maggiano, J. M., Fishman, M. (1983) 'Foveal lesions seen in retinitis pigmentosa.' *Archives of Ophthalmology*, **95**, 1993-1996.

Gartner, S., Henkind, P. (1982) 'Pathology of retinitis pigmentosa.' *Ophthalmology*, **89**, 1425-1432.

Harcourt, B., Hopkins, D. (1972) 'Tapetoretinal degeneration in childhood presenting as a disturbance of behaviour.' *British Medical Journal*, **1**, 202-205.

Hittner, H. M., Zeler, R. S. (1975) 'Ceroid-lipofuscinosis (Batten disease). Fluorescein angiography, electrophysiology, histopathology, ultrastructure, and a review of amaurotic familial idiocy.' *Archives of Ophthalmology*, **98**, 178-183.

Koerner, F., Schlote, W. (1972) 'Chronic progressive external ophthalmoplegia. Association with retinal pigmentary changes and evidence in favor of ocular myopathy.' *Archives of Ophthalmology,* **88,** 155-166.

Marmor, M. F., Aguirre, G., Arden, G., Berson, E., Birch, D. G., Boughman, J. A., Carr, R., Chatrian, G. E., Del Monte, M., Dowling, J., Enoch, J., Fishman, G. A., Fulton, A. B., Garcia, C. A., Gouras, P., Heckenlively, J., Hu, D., Lewis, R. A., Niemeyer, G., Parker, J. A., Perlman, I., Ripps, H., Sandberg, M. A., Siegel, I., Weleber, R. G., Wolf, M. L., Wu, L., Young, R. S. L. (1983) 'Retinitis pigmentosa. A symposium on terminology and methods of examination ' *Ophthalmology,* **90,** 126-131.

McKusick, V. A., Neufeld, E. F., Kelly, T. E. (1978) 'The mucopolysaccharide storage diseases.' *In* Stanbury, J. B., Wyngaarden, J. B., Fredrickson, D. S. (Eds.) *The Metabolic Basis of Inherited Disease, 4th Edn.* New York: McGraw-Hill. pp. 1282-1307.

Newell, F. W., Johnson, R. O., Huttenlocher, P. R. (1979) 'Pigmentary degeneration of the retina in the Hallervorden-Spatz syndrome.' *American Journal of Ophthalmology,* **88,** 467-471.

Noble, K. G., Carr, R. F. (1978) 'Leber's congenital amaurosis. A retrospective study of 33 cases and a histopathological study of one case.' *Archives of Ophthalmology,* **96,** 818-821.

Pearlman, J. T., Flood, T. P., Seiff, S. R. (1977) 'Retinitis pigmentosa without pigment.' *American Journal of Ophthalmology,* **81,** 417-419.

Peterson, W. S., Albert, D. M. (1974) 'Fundus changes in the hereditary nephropathie.' *Transactions of the American Academy of Ophthalmology and Otolaryngology,* **78,** 762-771.

Seiff, S. R., Heckenlively, J. R., Pearlman, J. T. (1982) 'Assessing the risk of retinitis pigmentosa with age-of-onset data.' *American Journal of Ophthalmology,* **94,** 38-43.

Yee, R. D., Herbert, P. N., Bergsma, D. R., Biemer, J. J. (1976) 'Atypical retinitis pigmentosa in familial hypobetalipoproteinemia.' *American Journal of Ophthalmology,* **82,** 64-71.

Cherry-red spot

Brownstein, S., Carpenter, S., Polomeno, R. C., Little, J. N. (1980) 'Sandnoff's disease (Gm$_2$ gangliosidosis type 2) histopathology and ultrastructure of the eye.' *Archives of Ophthalmology,* **98,** 1089-1097.

Cogan, D. G. (1966) 'Ocular correlates of inborn metabolic defects.' *Canadian Medical Association Journal,* **95,** 1055-1065.

Cogan, D. G., Chu, F. C., Gittinger, J., Tyschen, L. (1980) 'Fundal abnormalities of Gauchner's disease.' *Archives of Opthalmology,* **98,** 2202-2203.

Cotlier, E. (1971) 'Tay-Sachs' retina: deficiency of acetyl nexosaminidase A.' *Archives of Ophthalmology,* **86,** 352-356.

Emery, J. M., Green, W. R., Wyllie, R. G., Nowell, R. R. (1971) 'Gm$_1$-gangliosidosis, ocular and pathological manifestations.' *Archives of Ophthalmology,* **85,** 179-187.

Emery, J. M., Green, W. R., Huff, D. S., Sloan, H. R. (1972) 'Niemann-Pick disease (type C): histopathology and ultrastructure.' *American Journal of Ophthalmology,* **74,** 1144-1154.

Goldberg, M. F., Cotlier, E., Fichenscher, L. G., Kenyon, K., Enat, R., Borowsky, S. A. (1971) 'Macular cherry-red spot, corneal clouding, and β-galactosidase deficiency; clinical, biochemical, and electron microscopic study of a new autosomal recessive storage disease. *Archives of International Medicine,* **128,** 387-398.

Libert, J., Van Hoof, F., Toussaint, D., Roozitalab, H., Kenyon, K. P., Green, W. R. (1979) 'Ocular findings in metachromatic leukodystrophy. An electron microscopic and enzyme study in different clinical and genetic variants.' *Archives of Ophthalmology,* **97,** 1495-1504.

Rapin, I. (1976) 'Ocular correlates of inborn metabolic defects.' *Canadian Medical Association Journal,* **95,** 1055-1065.

Walton, D. S., Robb, R. M., Crocker, A. E. (1978) 'Ocular manifestations of group A Niemann-Pick disease.' *American Journal of Ophthalmology,* **85,** 174-180.

Macular degeneration

Barricks, M. E. (1977) 'Vitelliform lesions developing in normal fundi.' *American Journal of Ophthalmology,* **83,** 324-327.

Beckerman, B. L., Rapin, I. (1975) 'Ceroid lipofuscinosis.' *American Journal of Ophthalmology,* **80,** 73-77.

Carr, R. E., Noble, K. G. (1980) 'Juvenile macular degeneration.' *Ophthalmology,* **87,** 83-85.

Cibis, G. W., Morey, M., Harris, D. J. (1980) 'Dominantly inherited macular dystrophy with flecks (Stargardt).' *Archives of Ophthalmology,* **98,** 1785-1789.

Eagle, R. C., Lucier, A. C., Bernardino, V. B., Yanoff, M. (1980) 'Retinal pigment epithelial abnormalities in fundus flavimaculatus.' *Ophthalmology,* **87,** 1189-1200.

Gravina, R. F., Nakanishi, A. S., Faden, A. (1978) 'Subacute sclerosing panencephalitis.' *American Journal of Ophthalmology,* **86,** 106-109.

Hadden, O. B., Gass, J. D. M. (1976) 'Fundus flavimaculatus and Stargardt's disease.' *American Journal of Ophthalmology,* **82,** 527-539.
Krill, A. E. (1973) 'Juvenile macular degenerations. Part I.' *Ophthalmology Digest,* April 1973, 37-42.
Krill, A. E. (1973) 'Juvenile macular degnerations. Part II.' *Ophthalmology Digest,* May 1973, 33-40.
Krill, A. E., Morse, P. A., Potts, A. M., Klein, B. A. (1966) 'Hereditary vitelliform macular degeneration.' *American Journal of Ophthalmology,* **61,** 1405-1415.
Noble, K. G., Carr, R. (1979) 'Stargardt's disease and fundus flavimaculatus.' *Archives of Ophthalmology,* **97,** 1281-1285.
Schochet, S. S., Font, R. L., Morris, H. H. (1980) 'Jansky-Bielschowsky form of neuronal ceroid-lipofuscinosis.' *Archives of Ophthalmology,* **98,** 1083-1088.

Phakomata
Alexander, G. L., Norman, R. M. (1960) *The Sturge-Weber Syndrome.* Bristol: John Wright. pp. 1-87.
Cotlier, E. (1977) 'Cafe-au-lait spots of the fundus in neurofibromatosis.' *Archives of Ophthalmology,* **95,** 1990-1992.
Grover, W. D., Harley, R. D. (1969) 'Early recognition of tuberous sclerosis by funduscopic examination.' *Journal of Pediatrics,* **75,** 991-995.
Hardwig, P., Robertson, D. M. (1984) 'von Hippel-Lindau disease: a familial, often lethal multi-system phakomatosis.' *Ophthalmology,* **91,** 263-270.
Horowitz, P. (1971) 'von Hippel-Lindau disease.' *In* Tasman, W. (Ed.) *Retinal Diseases in Children.* New York: Harper & Row. pp. 78-91.
Kirby, T. J. (1951) 'Ocular phakomatoses.' *American Journal of Medical Sciences,* **222,** 227-239.
Lagos, J. C., Gomez, M. R. (1967) 'Tuberous sclerosis: reappraisal of a clinical entity.' *Mayo Clinical Proceedings,* **42,** 26-49.
Lewis, R. A., Riccardi, V. M. (1981) 'von Recklinghausen neurofibromatosis. Incidence of iris hamartomata.' *Ophthalmology,* **88,** 348-354.
Lloyd, L. A. (1973) 'Gliomas of the optic nerve and chiasma in childhood.' *Transactions of the American Ophthalmological Society,* **71,** 488-535.
Miller, S. J. H. (1963) 'Ophthalmic aspects of the Sturge-Weber syndrome.' *Proceedings of the Royal Society of Medicine,* **56,** 419-423.
Nyboer, J. H., Robertson, D. M., Gomez, M. R (1976) 'Retinal lesions in tuberous sclerosis.' *Archives of Ophthalmology,* **94,** 1277-1280.
Riley, F. C., Campbell, R. J. (1979) 'Double phakomatosis.' *Archives of Ophthalmology,* **97,** 518-520.
Salazar, F. G., Lamiell, J. M. (1980) 'Early identification of retinal angiomas in a large kindred with von Hippel-Lindau disease.' *American Journal of Ophthalmology,* **89,** 540-545.

Retinoblastoma
Char, D. H. (1980) 'Current concepts in retinoblastoma.' *Annals of Ophthalmology,* **12,** 792-804.
Dryja, T. P., Cavenee, W., White, R., Rapaport, J. M., Petersen, R., Albert, D. M., Bruns, G. A. P. (1984) 'Homozygosity of chromosome 13 in retinoblastoma.' *New England Journal of Medicine,* **310,** 550-553.
Gallie, B. L., Phillips, R. A. (1984) 'Retinoblastoma: a model of oncogenesis.' *Ophthalmology,* **91,** 666-672.
Howard, G. M., Ellsworth, R. M. (1965) 'Differential diagnosis of retinoblastoma. A statistical survey of 500 children. I. Relative frequency of the lesions which simulate retinoblastoma.' *American Journal of Ophthalmology,* **60,** 610-618.
Lopez, J. F.-V., Alvarez, J. C. (1983) 'Atypical echographic forms of retinoblastoma.' *Journal of Pediatric Ophthalmology and Strabismus,* **20,** 230-234.
Margo, C. E., Zimmerman, L. E. (1983) 'Retinoblastoma: the accuracy of clinical diagnosis in children treated by enucleation.' *Journal of Pediatric Ophthalmology and Strabismus,* **20,** 227-229.
Murphree, A. L., Benedict, W. F. (1984) 'Retinoblastoma: clues to human oncogenesis.' *Science,* **223,** 1028-1033.
Shields, J. A., Augsburger, J. J. (1981) 'Current approaches to the diagnosis and management of retinoblastoma.' *Survey of Ophthalmology,* **25,** 347-372.
Zimmerman, L. E., Burns, R. P., Wankum, G., Tully, R., Esterly, J. A. (1982) 'Trilateral retinoblastoma: ectopic intracranial retinoblastoma associated with bilateral retinoblastoma.' *Journal of Pediatric Ophthalmology and Strabismus,* **19,** 320-325.

Retinopathy of prematurity (retrolental fibroplasia)

Ashton, N. (1979) 'The pathogenesis of retrolental fibroplasia.' *Ophthalmology*, **86**, 1695-1699.

Brockhurst, R. J., Albert, D. M., Zakov, Z. N. (1981) 'Pathologic findings in familial exudative vitreoretinopathy.' *Archives of Ophthalmology*, **99**, 2143-2146.

Criswick, V. G., Schepens, C. L. (1969) 'Familial exudative vitreoretinopathy.' *American Journal of Ophthalmology*, **68**, 578-594.

Finer, N. N., Schindler, R. F., Peters, K. I., Grant, G. D. (1983) 'Vitamin E and retrolental fibroplasia. Improved visual outcome with early vitamin E.' *Ophthalmology*, **90**, 428-435.

Flynn, J. T., Cassady, J., Essner, D., Zeskind, J., Merritt, J., Flynn, R., Williams, M. J. (1979) 'Fluorescein angiography in retrolental fibroplasia: experience from 1969-1977.' *Ophthalmology*, **86**, 1700-1723.

Gow, J., Oliver, G. L. (1971) 'Familial exudative vitreoretinopathy. An expanded view.' *Archives of Ophthalmology*, **86**, 150-154.

Gunn, T. R., Easdown, J., Outerbridge, E. W., Aranda, J. V. (1980) 'Risk factors in retrolental fibroplasia.' *Pediatrics*, **65**, 1096-1100.

Palmer, E. A. (1981) 'Optimal timing of examination for acute retrolental fibroplasia.' *Ophthalmology*, **88**, 662-668.

Patz, A. (1983) 'Current therapy of retrolental fibroplasia, retinopathy of prematurity.' *Ophthalmology*, **90**, 425-427.

Schulman, J., Jampol, L. M., Schwartz, N. (1980) 'Peripheral proliferative retinopathy without oxygen therapy in a full-term infant.' *American Journal of Ophthalmology*, **90**, 509-514.

Slusher, M. M., Hutton, W. E. (1979) 'Familial exudative vitreoretinopathy.' *American Journal of Ophthalmology*, **87**, 152-156.

Tasman, W. (1979) 'Late complications of retrolental fibroplasia.' *Ophthalmology*, **86**, 1724-1740.

Hypertensive retinopathy

Tso, M. O. M., Jampol, L. M. (1982) 'Pathophysiology of hypertensive retinopathy.' *Ophthalmology*, **89**, 1132-1145.

Walsh, J. B. (1982) 'Hypertensive retinopathy. Description, classification and prognosis.' *Ophthalmology*, **89**, 1127-1131.

Diabetic retinopathy

Barr, C. C., Glaser, J. S., Blankenship, G. (1980) 'Acute disc swelling in juvenile diabetes. Clinical profile and natural history of 12 cases.' *Archives of Ophthalmology*, **98**, 2185-2192.

Frank, R. N., Hoffman, W. H., Podgor, M. J., Joondeph, H. C., Lewis, R. A., Margherio, R. R., Nachazel, D. P., Weiss, H., Christopherson, K. W., Cronin, M. A. (1980) 'Retinopathy in juvenile-onset diabetes of short duration.' *Ophthalmology*, **87**, 1-9.

Jackson, R. L., Ide, C. H., Guthrie, R. A., James, R. D. (1982) 'Retinopathy in adolescents and young adults with onset of insulin-dependent diabetes in childhood.' *Ophthalmology*, **89**, 7-13.

Noble, K. G., Carr, R. E. (1983) 'Diabetic retinopathy. I. Nonproliferative retinopathy.' *Ophthalmology*, **90**, 1261-1263.

Lipemia retinalis

Kurz, G. H., Shakib, M., Sohmer, K. K., Friedman, A. H. (1976) 'The retina in type 5 hyperlipoproteinemia.' *American Journal of Ophthalmology*, **82**, 32-43.

Vinger, P. F., Sachs, B. A. (1970) 'Ocular manifestations of hyperlipoproteinemia.' *American Journal of Ophthalmology*, **70**, 563-573.

Roth spots

Duane, T. D., Osher, R. H., Green, W. R. (1980) 'White centered hemorrhages: their significance.' *Ophthalmology*, **87**, 66-69.

Phelps, C. D. (1971) 'The association of pale-centered retinal hemorrhages with intracranial bleeding in infancy.' *American Journal of Ophthalmology*, **72**, 348-350.

Leukemic retinopathy

Allen, R. A., Straatsma, B. R. (1961) 'Ocular involvement in leukemia and allied disorders.' *Archives of Ophthalmology*, **66**, 490-508.

Chalfin, A. I., Nash, B. M., Goldstein, J. H. (1973) 'Optic nervehead involvement in lymphocytic leukemia.' *Journal of Pediatric Ophthalmology*, **10**, 39-43.

Holt, J. M., Gordon-Smith, E. C. (1969) 'Retinal abnormalities in diseases of the blood.' *British Journal of Ophthalmology*, **53**, 145-160.

Ridgeway, E. W., Jaffe, N., Walton, D. S. (1976) 'Leukemic ophthalmopathy in children.' *Cancer*, **38**, 1744-1749.

Rosenthal, A. R. (1983) 'Ocular manifestations of leukemia.' *Ophthalmology*, **90**, 899-905.

79

Retinal telangiectasis

Archer, D. B. (1971) 'Leber's miliary aneurysms.' *Ophthalmology Digest,* July 1971, 8-13.

Farkas, T. G., Potts, A. M., Boone, C. (1973) Some pathologic and biochemical aspects of Coats' disease.' *American Journal of Ophthalmology,* **75,** 289-301.

Gass, J. D. M. (1971) 'Cavernous hemangioma of the retina: a neuro-cutaneous syndrome.' *American Journal of Ophthalmology,* **71,** 799-814.

Gass, J. D., Oyakawaw, R. T. (1982) 'Idiopathic juxtafoveolar retinal telangiectasis.' *Archives of Ophthalmology,* **100,** 769-780.

Goldberg, R. E., Pheasant, T. R., Shields, J. A. (1979) 'Cavernous hemangioma of the retina. A four-generation pedigree with neurocutaneous manifestations and an example of bilateral retinal involvement.' *Archives of Ophthalmology,* **97,** 2321-2324.

Reese, A. B. (1956) 'Telangiectasis of the retina and Coat's disease.' *American Journal of Ophthalmology,* **42,** 1-8.

Retinal arteriolar tortuosity

Goldberg, M. F., Pollack, I. P., Green, W. R. (1972) 'Familial retinal arteriolar tortuosity with retinal hemorrhage.' *American Journal of Ophthalmology,* **73,** 183-191.

Prepapillary vascular loops

Brown, G. C., Magargal, L., Augsburger, J. J., Shields, J. A. (1979) 'Preretinal arterial loops and retinal arterial occlusion.' *American Journal of Ophthalmology,* **87,** 646-651.

Degenhart, W., Brown, G. C., Augsburger, J. J., Magargal, L. (1981) 'Prepapillary vascular loops. A clinical and fluorescein angiographic study.' *Ophthalmology,* **88,** 1126-1131.

Albinotic fundus

Bergsma, D. R., Kaiser-Kupfer, M. (1974) 'A new form of albinism.' *American Journal of Ophthalmology,* **77,** 837-844.

Creel, D., O'Donnell, F. E., Witkop, C. J. (1978) 'Visual system anomalies in human ocular albinos.' *Science,* **102,** 931-933.

diGeorge, A. M., Ounsted, R. W., Harley, R. D. (1960) 'Waardenburg syndrome.' *Journal of Pediatrics,* **57,** 649-669.

Falls, H. F. (1953) 'Albinism.' *Transactions of the American Academy of Ophthalmology and Otolaryngology,* **57,** 324-331.

Hittner, H. M., King, R. A., Riccardi, V. M., Ledbetter, D. H., Borda, R. P., Ferrell, R. E., Kretzer, F. L. (1982) 'Oculocutaneous albinoidism as a manifestation of reduced neural crest derivatives in the Prader-Willi syndrome.' *American Journal of Ophthalmology,* **94,** 328-337.

O'Donnell, F. E., Hambrick, G. W., Green, W. R., Iliff, W. J., Stone, D. L. (1976) 'X-linked ocular albinism. An oculocutaneous macromelanosomal disorder.' *Archives of Ophthalmology,* **94,** 1883-1892.

O'Donnell, F. E., King, R. A., Green, W. R., Witkop, C. J. (1978) 'Autosomal recessively inherited ocular albinism. A new form of ocular albinism affecting females as severely as males.' *Archives of Ophthalmology,* **96,** 1621-1626.

Simon, J. W., Adams, R. J., Calhoun, J. H., Shapiro, S. S., Ingerman, C. M. (1982) 'Ophthalmic manifestations of the Hermansky-Pudlak syndrome (oculocutaneous albinism and hemorrhagic diathesis).' *American Journal of Ophthalmology,* **93,** 71-77.

Fundus albipunctatus

Carr, R. E., Margolis, S., Siegel, I. M. (1984) 'Fluorescein angiography and vitamin A and oxalate levels in fundus albipunctatus.' *American Journal of Ophthalmology,* **82,** 549-558.